Intensive Care

Suzanne Crowe grew up in Bray, County Wicklow, and studied medicine at Trinity College Dublin. She went on to train in anaesthesiology and intensive care medicine and practises mostly with children.

She is currently a consultant in paediatric intensive-care medicine at Children's Health Ireland in Crumlin, Ireland's largest acute paediatric teaching hospital, and president of the Irish Medical Council. She has a passionate interest in children's rights, especially in terms of health and social care, sits on several charity boards including LGBT Ireland and Cheshire Ireland, and has a regular column in the *Irish Independent* in which she writes about healthcare and child-related topics.

She is a widow with five children, one of whom – Beatrice – died shortly after she was born. Beatrice was Suzanne's major inspiration to work in intensive care for children.

Suzanne lives in Dublin. *Intensive Care* is her first book.

Intensive Care

True Stories of Healing, Heartache and Hope from Inside Irish Children's Medicine

Dr Suzanne Crowe

HACHETTE
BOOKS
IRELAND

First published in Ireland in 2025 by
HACHETTE BOOKS IRELAND

1

Cataloguing in Publication Data is available from the British Library

ISBN 9781399741064

Typeset in Berling LT Std by Palimpsest Book Production Ltd,
Falkirk, Stirlingshire

Printed and bound in Great Britain by
Clays Ltd, Elcograf S.p.A.

Hachette Books Ireland policy is to use papers that are natural, renewable
and recyclable products and made from wood grown in sustainable forests.
The logging and manufacturing processes are expected to conform to the
environmental regulations of the country of origin.

MIX
Paper | Supporting
responsible forestry
FSC
www.fsc.org
FSC® C104740

Hachette Books Ireland
8 Castlecourt Centre
Castleknock
Dublin 15, Ireland
(info@hbgi.ie)

Authorised representative in the EEA

A division of Hachette UK Ltd
Carmelite House, 50 Victoria Embankment, London EC4Y 0DZ

www.hachettebooksireland.ie

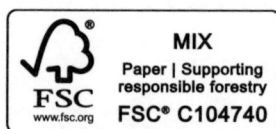

To anyone whose life has been changed by
their love for a child

Author's Note

I began writing this book several years ago after I gave a speech in the College of Anaesthesiologists, which recounted a memorable young patient and the unique care that a colleague had given them. A number of people present found the story moving, and suggested that I capture some of my experiences for a wider audience.

During the time of writing, issues around the funding, organisation and delivery of children's health services have come sharply into focus in Ireland. This focus is welcome and should result in substantial improvement. Children have no vote and pay no tax. The consequences of decisions made on their behalf can be lifelong, seeping through generations of families.

There is a deep well of compassion and love for children in our health service. I believe this book speaks to that and gives a sense of hope to where we find ourselves.

1. Casting the Die

'Wisdom begins in wonder.'

Socrates

A doctor is often asked why they chose their path in life. On tough days it's a question you ask yourself. Everyone has their reasons. As a teenager, I was heading towards writing or art after school, but something happened that changed my direction, though I didn't realise its impact at the time.

Even before I veered towards becoming a doctor, though, one of my early memories is of my mother propping up my youngest sister, Louise, to breathe. I was nine years old. We were wild with excitement when our little sister arrived, a gap of seven years between this gorgeous baby girl and the rest of us. But at five weeks old, she got whooping cough. Too young to be immunised, she was vulnerable to infection. Dr Kelly, our GP, diagnosed it when my mother brought her to him: she was coughing so much, she couldn't keep milk down.

Sitting in the kitchen with Louise on her lap, my mother would hold her upright when she started coughing. She cupped the baby's head in her hand and tapped her gently on the back. She would count how many seconds of silence had passed with our baby sister not breathing – until finally, with little blue lips, she took in a loud, whoopy breath. The silence waiting for her next breath was terrifying. Even as children we knew that something very bad was happening. It went on for days and nights.

'If we get to sixty seconds, I'll run across to Dr Kelly with her,' my mother would say to us each time Louise had a coughing spell. My father shook his head silently.

'I'll run with you, Mammy,' I said. 'I can run fast.'

'I'll be out and gone if she stops,' my mother said, one eye on the closed kitchen door. Terror clutched at my heart.

I'll run with you, I repeated, in my head.

Louise recovered and grew into a wonderful woman.

My resolve to run and help became my purpose.

2. Mrs Johnson

'All genuine learning comes through experience.'
John Dewey

Each person working in health and social care has their own reasons for choosing to do so. We humans are walking, talking, breathing ten-thousand-piece jigsaws. We carry fragments of life events, chunky pieces of the people who have cared about us and splinters of those who didn't care enough. Our choices are complicated.

Several events in my school years shook me to the core. Each generated the same feeling of intense helplessness. Each forged an enduring connection to another's pain. Those overwhelming emotions directed me towards becoming a doctor. It took me many years to see that.

When I was fifteen, my school embarked on its first transition year. I told my mother I wasn't going to do it as I needed to leave school as quickly as possible.

'Grand,' she said. My mother is an extremely wise woman.

Then she went to a meeting at the school. When she came home, she said, 'Sister Kathleen says you're to do this

3

new transition year.' And so it was decided. Sister Kathleen was a formidable headmistress, and I didn't stand a chance in a head-to-head with her, especially if she now had my mother on her side. It turned out to be a fantastic year of growth and fun. Along with many other activities, we did two work-experience placements.

First I went to a graphic-design studio in a huge tumble-down Georgian house, run by two totally relaxed artists in woolly sweaters and jeans. It was a wonderful week, making tea, eating chocolate digestives, painting logos and taking photographs. Both men encouraged my interest in art and gave pointers on applying for art courses after I'd left school. Jonas, the quieter of the pair, offered to help put together my portfolio over the summer of fifth year.

The second week of work experience was intended to have a social or community aspect to it. My placement was on the female surgical ward of our local hospital, where the nurses had never before encountered a secondary-school student on a ward and didn't really know what to do with me. My main tasks that the nursing staff came up with that week were helping older patients eat their lunch, making beds with a chatterbox student nurse called Melissa and changing bedpans. On the fourth day, an older nurse, rushing past me, pointed at a curtain around a bed and said, 'Go in to Mrs Johnson and take her off the bedpan.'

I went to the bed and pulled back the curtain. I was queen of the bedpans at that stage, all week whipping them out of the bed and carrying them quick-smart to the sluice for emptying and cleaning. Patients were usually just waking up after surgery but were able to lift their hips and generally looked grateful, or almost as embarrassed as I felt. But it felt good to be useful.

That day, something different was going on behind the thin blue curtain. Mrs Johnson was a tiny old lady, her lined face as white as the pillow behind her head. She looked extremely sick to me, with my newly acquired knowledge of patients in hospital. As I peered at her in the gloom cast by the curtain, I wondered if she was dead. 'Mrs Johnson, I'm here to take your bedpan out,' I whispered. She opened her eyes but said nothing, and closed them again.

Well, I'd better get on with it, I thought, remembering the somewhat scary nurse who had commanded me to do the job.

I pulled back the old lady's blankets. What I saw left me feeling faint and for a couple of moments the room spun, waves of nausea crashing down on my head. I did not know that Mrs Johnson had had both of her legs amputated earlier that day, above her knees. In fact, I didn't even know that it was possible to have both of your legs removed by surgeons and still be alive, in a hospital bed, on the female surgical ward.

Skin-coloured bandages were wrapped around her upper thighs, with blood oozing through the bandages in places. Two drains hung into the bed beside the stumps of her legs, with clots in the bottles connected to the drains.

She must have heard me whimper in terror because she opened her eyes and looked at my horrified face as, transfixed, I stared at her legs. I was stuck to the spot. Neither of us said anything. She started to cry. She cried like a five-year-old child, scared and left alone in the world. To my shame, I stepped away from her bed and pulled the curtain closed.

I stood behind the curtain, in shock, the thin nylon gripped in my hands. My head swam. I thought I could smell blood. I probably couldn't but I believed I could. It smelt like the butcher's on the main street in the town where my mother went each Saturday.

The elderly lady continued to cry. I realised I couldn't walk away, yet I had nothing to offer her. I went back behind the curtain, sat down in the plastic chair beside her bed, took her hand and she wept for what felt like hours. I chewed my lip silently, swallowing hard. I was fifteen; she was seventy-five. I understand now, as an adult, that we all long to be cared for, and that that longing for care is entangled with our ability to be caregivers. Our common human frailty leads to empathy.

At the end of the afternoon, when it was time to catch the bus home, that senior nurse asked me was I OK. I said yes, which wasn't quite true. She apologised for sending me in to Mrs Johnson on my own. 'That's all right,' I replied. 'It was good to be able to help.' That week no one encouraged me to consider a job in a hospital. By Friday, they all seemed tired, and I was more exhausted than I had ever been.

Mrs Johnson is long gone from this world, but she is one of the jigsaw pieces that are part of me now. Each piece represents a person, and their investment in my life, known or unknown to them. When I sit in the paediatric intensive-care unit, where I now work, with distressed mothers and fathers, sometimes I see a glimpse of their five-year-old selves, feeling such pain and wondering why this horrible thing has happened, wondering who will care for them. I reassure them that we will care for them and that we will try to help with the pain. Often I pause to remember and thank Mrs Johnson.

3. A Stone in My Shoe

'Let the waves carry you where the light cannot.'
Mohit Kaushik

When I was three years old my family moved to Bray to get away from the spreading city of Dublin. My father continued to work in the city, rising early in the morning and leaving on the bus with the sandwiches my mother had packed. We never did outrun the city completely, but Bray was a wonderful place to grow up. It had a small-town feel, with the bonus of being seaside.

We spent many days on the stony beach, swimming, chasing each other and searching for treasure among the debris washed up by the tide. On the shelf above my bed, I had a box of pebbles collected from the shoreline, kept for their colour or their shape. One of five children, I was a day-dreamer. As a young child I'd hide in a nest of cushions behind the sofa with a book in my hand. Stories filled my growing mind and, through them, I travelled to every corner of the world. My father bought us the *Childcraft* encyclopedia – all twelve volumes of it – and we leapfrogged from there to more advanced books. Reading was nourishment and solace.

I went to the local girls' secondary school, a convent run by the Loreto nuns. There, I had a positive experience of education, with a strong flavour of female empowerment fostered by the principal. With Sr Kathleen at the helm, there were debating teams, public-speaking prizes, quizzes, business projects, science fairs and model government groups. In that rich environment, I flourished and considered pursuing my love of words or art as a career. But early experiences with sick people, like Mrs Johnson, were as tiny stones in my shoe. Quietly but relentlessly they pulled my attention in their direction, until I switched my ambition to becoming a doctor. At the time, I didn't make the connection consciously, but it was a source of worry for my mother when, as a teenager, I began to talk about studying medicine.

With five children in our family, we didn't have much money, although my dad had a good trade as a compositor with the *Irish Press* newspaper. He worked as much overtime as he could. He took night shifts for weeks on end, and as a result my mother was the *tour de force* in keeping everything together. 'Don't worry,' she said, whenever I raised the question about university fees and years of study. We were deep in the 1980s recession in Ireland so university fees and a prolonged college lifestyle were out of reach of most people. 'You get the marks, and I'll find the money.' Then she'd laugh, and say, 'I might have the easier job! You'd better get back upstairs to those books.'

But it wasn't just the money. Neither of my parents had gone to university and it was seen as a different world. No one knew anyone who had successfully navigated their way into medical school, apart from our GP. Information about going to university was obtained from libraries, teachers and the post office. We had to apply to the county council for a financial grant, my mother sending my father to work with requests for letters about tax and payslips. We deliberated over the endless forms and eventually posted them as the Leaving Certificate exams crept closer.

My mother engaged in the new activity of finding other people in the town who had successfully got a grant to go to college. She would relay updates to me when I came downstairs from studying, to take a break and watch *Coronation Street* with her. 'We've every reason to be hopeful,' she declared one evening, after regaling me, in detail, with the story of a man called Cearbhall O'Dalaigh. He was a Bray legend, the son of a fishmonger who had studied law and become Chief Justice of Ireland. Never shy of telling a tale or two, she made this great man sound completely relatable, as though he had grown up next door to us. 'And if the grant application doesn't work, I'll find another way,' she concluded.

Her indefatigable optimism made me laugh. I suggested I could defer for a year or two, if I was offered a place. I could get a job and save money to start the course.

'Oh, no,' my mother said firmly. 'If you get a place, you'll go straight away. We didn't get those kinds of chances,' she continued, in a softer voice, referring to herself and my dad. She paused, looking at the television rather than at me. I stayed quiet. She came back to me after a moment or so. 'Life doesn't give you chances very often. You've got to go now.

'It will be worth the sacrifices.'

As summer came to an end, I was offered a place to read medicine at Trinity College Dublin, based on my examination results. The shiny apple of ambition hung tantalisingly just out of reach. I knew my parents would lift me up to take a bite.

A few days after the exam results had been released, the Royal College of Surgeons in Ireland called me for an interview for a full scholarship to study medicine. If I won it, the scholarship would change everything at home.

My grandfather brought me into the city for the interview. It was a gorgeous August afternoon as he parked on St Stephen's Green. I had never had an interview for anything before and had not known how to prepare for it. At my mother's suggestion, I wore a navy skirt suit and white blouse, my older sister's uniform, which she wore working in a bank.

In the front hall of RCSI, my grandfather stopped to chat to every single person, telling each one that we had never been in this imposing building before and that his granddaughter was going to be a doctor. I was mortified, of course, but the pride in his voice was a gift.

A woman ushered me into a long hall. Eight strangers sat behind a table and I peered at them through the muted light cast by windows high above my head. The strangers appeared to be miles away as I walked the length of the hall, my shoes squeaking on the ancient wooden boards. I was trying to breathe slowly and seem calm. Huge oil paintings of men from hundreds of years ago hung on the walls.

An elderly man with a kind face and a deep voice welcomed me and invited me to sit on the solitary chair opposite the table. The interview passed quickly and felt surprisingly pleasant as I relaxed into their curiosity and conversation. The only question I can recall was one man asked why I had chosen art as a subject for my exams and wondered who my favourite artist was. I talked about the drawing classes my mother had brought me to as a small child and the work of Pauline Bewick, which I adored.

As I stood up to leave, my heart thumped painfully as it occurred to me that we hadn't spoken anything about being a doctor. I felt so young and silly.

'How did it go?' asked my grandfather, anxiously, when I emerged back into the warm sunny street.

I shrugged. 'It was OK, I think.'

The following day, my mum answered the phone to a woman from the admissions office.

'Oh. Oh, that's wonderful!' I heard her say. But then silence.

'Oh, no.' Another silence.

'Is there no chance?' she asked.

There was silence in the kitchen as my mother stood listening to the woman at the other end.

'I see. Thank you. We'll have to think about this.' My mum sounded serious now. A tiny bit sad, even.

Louise ran into the kitchen with her little friend from across the street. Their excited shouts about a dog running on the road distracted us for a moment. I waited for my mum to tell me what the woman from RCSI had said. I had been awarded a place to study. But not a scholarship.

'It's fine,' she said. 'It's fine,' she repeated, but I knew she was disappointed. 'You're still going to do this,' she said. 'We will not let it stop us.'

A couple of days later, a letter from Wicklow County Council arrived, containing a grant offer to cover my fees for six years at Trinity College Dublin. My mother was right. I was going to study medicine and become a doctor. The way ahead was clear: success at university, become a skilful surgeon, find a partner and have a family, travel the world and be content in that life. There is a proverb about making God laugh by telling him your dreams – little did I know what was in store.

But even more than that, little did I know how much that life would change me as a person, and as a doctor. The two became inextricable.

4. Adrift

'One has to decide whether one's fears or one's hopes are what should matter most.'

Atul Gawande

By the end of second year, I'd made up my mind. Medicine was not for me. The days of lectures and laboratory work-shops were long, stuffed full of biochemistry, physiology, anatomy and statistics. I found it difficult to connect the work with helping people.

I was failing anatomy, which triggered what was called a 'pass/fail viva', a practical, spoken examination in the presence of two lecturers in the subject. I bumped my way through it, scraping a pass mark. But instead of proceeding joyfully to the pub to celebrate, I found myself in the senior tutor's office, with breaking news.

'I want to leave medicine,' I told him.

The professor was a quiet man with a kind face. He sighed gently. 'It's very common to take a while to settle into your subject.'

'I hate it,' I replied, with a touch of teenager petulance.

I was turning twenty shortly. 'It's nothing like I thought it would be.'

'What course are you thinking of changing to?' he asked.

'English,' I replied, ready to argue my case.

'How will that serve you better? It won't be what you think it will be either.' He paused, and smiled with his eyes. 'That is the essential nature of life. It is nothing like you think it is.'

After another ten minutes or so of chat, Professor Ignatius McGovern concluded our meeting with the vague commitment that he would 'look into it over the summer. Come back to me in September, and we'll see how to change your subject.'

As he walked me down the dark, austere steps of the physics building his parting words to me were, 'See what changes you could make yourself in the meantime. I imagine you have the tools of change right there inside you.'

He was right. The tools of change were there, to re-frame the challenges and to add much-needed patience. The course was difficult because it was meant to be difficult.

I returned to medicine at the start of the third year. Our subjects became more patient-focused that year, and within a matter of months our class had made the move to hospital life. The shift in focus from dusty books to real people was a turning point. The early clinical years of learning to listen to people and examine their bodies are precious building blocks to which a doctor returns again and again. Like the beads on a rosary, the mind of a doctor is shaped through endless repetition of the sequence: listen, observe, examine, reflect, act. Repeat. Those steps quickly become innate.

They are the mental tools to be applied to the problems people bring to you. Those people are your patients.

My class and I had wonderful teachers when we were learning to be doctors. Most of them taught in a haphazard, slightly frantic style, as they dashed between their own clinical duties. They shared a crazy passion for their work, which was electrifying to encounter as a student.

Life in hospital was shockingly raw, and strangely addictive. I spent an increasing amount of time on the wards and in the operating rooms, clinging to the guidance and self-deprecating humour of older doctors. They wore their experiences in a weary, resigned fashion that dissolved into laughter when they were in the doctors' lounge. No one ever spoke of how they felt about anything. It was *M*A*S*H*, it was *ER*. We would be doctors, and we would be tough.

At the same time, life changed at home.

5. Fading Away

'We love life, not because we are used to living, but because we are used to loving.'

Friedrich Nietzsche

Austin was my grandfather. Well, his name was Augustine, but he was only ever known in our family as Austin or Granddad. We had several generations of men and women who were christened with one name and called another. He was a retired postman and lived with us after Granny died. He was a wonderful carpenter and teacher. He taught me how to drive, in his silver VW Polo, insisting that I got to know the engine before I was even allowed to put on my seatbelt. To this day, I have an odd affection for engines and cars. As teenagers growing up with him in the house, he drove us crazy with his conservative views and plodding ways. But he was loved deeply, because of and despite the things that made us rage at him.

He was desperately proud when we discovered that I was going to medical school and would become a doctor. Before we left for my interview at RCSI, we checked the engine oil and water, then made sure the tyres were firm. We were travelling ten kilometres there and back, and he insisted we should be certain that the car was up to this important task.

For years he had been shuttling back and forth every six months into St Vincent's Hospital where he would spend a day displaying various clinical signs and regaling the medical students with stories. 'They can't find out why my fingers are like this!' he would marvel to anyone within earshot. 'None of the doctors know why they're all swollen, and they're very clever in there.'

My grandfather had what I later learnt is called 'clubbing'. His fingertips were bulbous, with the nailbeds splayed across the top. They had been like that for as long as any of us could remember, and as he was still able to make anything he wanted from wood, he wasn't bothered by them. He revelled in the days out with the UCD students and would come home in the Polo with as many tall tales about them as, no doubt, he had told them. Granddad enjoyed people, and he liked being the centre of attention.

By the time I had reached the clinical years of medical study, two things had changed: I had learnt that clubbing can be a sign of lung cancer. And Granddad had passed away from lung cancer and liver metastasis. In the months before, he'd begun to look a bit thin. He'd never carried much weight, but he became slight. Then his eyes went yellow. My mother sent him up to the GP, who sent him into the hospital. They didn't keep him long, just a few days. In retrospect I understand why the brief stay.

I was twenty-one and coming to the end of my first three years in medicine, which I had found terribly difficult. Not only because of the mounting study but also because the subjects weren't as exciting as I had expected. I would never be even close to top of the class, always felt behind and had boyfriend troubles. Caught up in my own head, it was a couple of weeks before I saw what my parents could see: my grandfather was softly fading away, like dusky evening light in a clear sky.

No one said anything about cancer, until one day, my mother whispered to me urgently, 'Your granddad doesn't know that he has cancer. So don't say anything. It will only upset him.' So now I knew.

In our family, cancer had been feared for generations, although we didn't know many people who had had it. Everyone was terrified of it. It was unspeakable. My granny had perpetuated the dread throughout her years of avoiding any doctor of any kind for fear that they might say the word 'cancer'. It was only ever whispered as 'The Big C', if it had to be mentioned at all. Sadly, she had uncontrolled hypertension and diabetes and died relatively young from a devastating stroke.

On a Sunday afternoon towards the end of his life, Granddad left the dinner table and went into the sitting room. My mother was tidying up and I stood to help her. 'Go and sit inside with your granddad,' she said, in a way that wasn't looking for a discussion.

In the sitting room, Granddad sat upright in a dining chair, breathing with deliberation. Not panting or huffing, but each breath seemed carefully chosen to follow the previous one. I sat opposite him and smiled encouragingly. Minutes passed without us talking.

'I'm going to die soon,' Granddad said matter-of-factly, looking directly into my eyes. He saw my alarmed face. 'I'm not afraid. I've lived enough now. Your mother thinks I don't know that I have cancer,' he continued. 'Of course I know. Isn't it in *my* body?' he added, with a more forceful and impatient breath.

A few moments of silence passed.

'You're going to meet lots of people like me,' he said, almost with an air of satisfaction. 'People who have cancer.'

I couldn't think of a single word to say back to him, but he didn't seem to mind. He was on a mission to say his piece.

'I want you to remember that those people who have the cancer ...' he paused to catch his breath a bit '... they are the same as me. Do you understand?' he asked.

I shook my head. 'No.'

'They are granddads, and dads, and mams, and sisters,' he replied. 'They are not just cancer.'

I nodded vigorously to show I'd heard him.

'And they always know they have the cancer.' He winked as he said this, smiling a little sadly. 'Don't worry if you can't fix them. Just be kind and help them keep their dignity.'

He closed his eyes and seemed to doze for a while. I flicked on the TV and watched a bit of football. Liverpool was playing Ipswich. The room was warm as sunshine streamed through the patio doors. I felt quite snoozy myself.

'I always liked living here with you lot.' Granddad spoke again. 'Won't you make sure your brothers and sisters know I'm very grateful to them for making space for me?' he said, gesturing around the room with his hand, as if we were all there right now, and shuffling across on the sofa. 'And your dad. Not easy for your dad to have another man in the house.'

And that was it. He had said what was on his mind, closed his eyes again and made loud, manly snores, his head leaning against the chair back.

Within a month or so he was gone. Just as he had said he would be. I'm the one now who feels grateful. Grateful for knowing a simple man without secrets, a person with pride, who spoke sparingly and comfortably showed love by teaching those he loved.

He taught me about cars because it created a bridge between us. Such almost inconsequential connections between people open a door to trust and a deeper understanding.

In my own practice of medicine, I listen to the story that is woven around the illness. A child may fall off a bouncy castle at a christening party in a garden that adjoins another garden. That garden has a pond. The neighbour runs in to help . . . Each detail in the story is added by the patient for a reason. It can take some time to figure out why certain details are important, which ones have a factual element to them, and which have an emotion associated with them. With trust and confidence, we uncover the reasons together. I genuinely believe that every single detail matters. The 'why' may come many years later.

My grandfather taught me to see the person, not the illness.

6. Setting Out

*'You have to be willing to go to war with yourself and
create a whole new identity.'*

David Goggins

In the hospital years of training, I loved meeting patients.
If I felt shy, I imagined my mother was with me and how
easily she would chat to people. The generosity of patients,
who shared their stories and their illnesses with us as
students, was extraordinary.

I gravitated towards surgery, especially enjoying the
atmosphere in the operating room. I hung around the
department of surgery and operating rooms all the time,
listening intently to the attitude and language used by those
who worked in that special place. The joy of a task achieved,
individually and as a team, was obvious.

As a team, the surgeons had a strong professional identity,
which they reinforced at every opportunity. 'We are
surgeons' was a frequent reply to any number of questions.
'We are surgeons' explained their demanding drive for
perfection from themselves and everyone in their orbit.

Over time, my gaze shifted to the anaesthesiologists. Their cool, controlled grasp on the ebb and flow of each case fascinated me. During an operation, the surgeons focused on the part of the patient's body that required correction. It seemed to me, as a student, that the anaesthesiologist steadily held the entire patient and the team. They exuded a different kind of confidence from the surgeons. They were eerily calm, the kind of calm that came from years of managing the wide variety of cases that are thrust upon them. They acquired the skills and knowledge to catalogue risk, anticipate it, prioritise it correctly and manage it well in advance of any event occurring. To an outsider watching an anaesthesiologist working, they would believe that nothing was happening. It was the very opposite of helplessness. That was where I wanted to be.

In the basement of the hospital where we were allocated residence, there were two tiny library rooms. My fellow students and I spent every hour we could there in the weeks before our final exams. We surfaced only to be fed by the generous ladies in the hospital canteen.

At home at weekends, I practised my clinical examination on my youngest sister, Louise, who was then ten years old. She patiently sat while I performed structured examination routines to elucidate signs of illness, speaking the names of eponymous syndromes into the air above her head. She was sometimes joined by our neighbour's child. Although they made faces and giggled at each other, from my stern face they knew better than to interrupt my flow of Latin phrases and lists of pathologies.

The day after the final exam results were pinned to a noticeboard in the medical school, my parents came in. Our plan was to see the results and go for lunch together. They already knew that I had passed my final medical exams, but they wanted to read them for themselves. My father insisted on reading the complete class list of names and results aloud. They were listed in order of merit. When he came to my name, he swallowed and paused.

My mother began to cry softly, turning her face into my father's jacket, looking like a young girl beside his tall frame. Then she hugged me and thanked me, for making one of her dreams come true. The woman who made everything happen humbly gave me her gratitude.

Years later, when a parent thanked me for what we had done to help their child, I had the same sense of swimming in a sea of indebtedness. I was grateful to them for the fulfilment their child had given me. They were grateful to me for the care. We swam together.

7. Taking a History

'After nourishment, shelter and companionship, stories are the thing we need most in the world.'
                                        Philip Pullman

On graduation in 1995, I worked as an intern in the Meath and Adelaide hospitals in Dublin, then began structured training as an anaesthesiologist. That training brought me through a dozen different hospitals and seven years of my life. Those years passed in the blink of an eye, with thousands of hours on duty in the hospital, more exams and plenty of nights out, dancing and laughing.

I shared a house in the city centre with friends and we had a lot of parties. When we were not on call in the hospital or out in a nightclub, we were curled up on the sofa swapping stories about friends, our families and our patients. Sick people and what had happened to them occupied our minds endlessly. Medicine is an oral art, originally an apprenticeship, with the learning gained from each other through the medium of stories. Patients tell us their stories. We tell those stories to each other.

The stories have immense power. The phrases used, the words left unsaid. When we first meet a patient, we ask a set of questions that is drummed into us at medical school. The questions change a little, depending on the particular area of medicine in which we're working. This is called 'taking a history'. We take the patient's story and craft a narrative to explain their symptoms and direct us towards treatment. Listening carefully for specific details trains your ear and teaches you to observe body language closely.

But, of course, patients don't know which details you're searching for, so they tell their stories in the way they want to tell them, in a fashion that makes sense to them. This is where the magic lies, being present, listening to the seeds of trust being planted. It is an enormous privilege to hear people's stories. It is even more an honour to carry them forward, to ensure that they mean almost as much to others as they do to the patient.

People often make the mistake of believing that an anaesthesiologist or intensive-care doctor spends all their time with patients who are sleeping and that they miss out on hearing their stories. This is far from true.

In the operating department, the small room where a patient is anaesthetised has the atmosphere of a quiet confessional. As a doctor beginning my training in anaesthesia, I noticed this straight away. Waiting for my supervising consultant to join us, I would frequently chat to patients about their lives, having already carried out my medical assessment on the ward. Patients are often quite nervous as they get closer to surgery, and gentle conversation is helpful for some.

I recall one young man who arrived at the anaesthesia room chained to a prison guard. We chatted about the weather and football, before I noticed his date of birth. 'Oh, we were born on the same day!' I remarked to him.

'Were you born in Dublin, Doctor?' he asked me.

'Yes, I was.' I smiled. 'What a funny thought, that we were born at the same time, same city,' I went on.

'Yeah,' he said, after a moment. 'But I wasn't born to be a doctor.'

The prison guard laughed in a nasty tone, designed to remind all of us of our place.

I fell silent. I felt sad and awkward, as if I had been rude and broken a boundary between us. Sensing how uncomfortable I was, the patient spoke again: 'Yer mam and dad must be very proud of you, being a doctor an' all.'

Even now, decades later, this man's sensitivity to my feelings and his kindness brings a tear to my eyes. I wasn't born to be a doctor. Nor was he. He wasn't born to be in a prison either. We had different starts in life. That was all. My parents lifted me into the opportunities I was lucky enough to be offered. Had I stumbled, they would have lifted me a second time or a third. The young man I met had stumbled, tempted as a teenager into trouble. His home life lacked the capacity to lift him up and guide him onwards.

The potential of every child and the importance of childhood is a theme running through many of our patients' stories, even when they are very old, when their story is told backwards. It makes the care of children vitally important, each child a seed of the adult, to be nourished and loved.

8. Nights with No Sleep

'True terror isn't being scared; it's not having a choice on the matter.'

John Green

It was during the whirlwind of moving training jobs every three or six months that I met my future husband, Barry. We were at a Christmas party, hosted by friends of friends. It was 1998. He had recently returned to Dublin after a decade of working in investment banking in London. I think he always had a romantic thing for doctors, and he adored the strange life we lived.

We fell in love. Very quickly Barry had a vision of what our life would be as a couple and as a family. He settled in and prepared to wait with a persistence that intrigued me. After six months of dating, Barry suggested we buy a house together, as it made 'good financial sense'. Studying for yet another anaesthesiology exam, I agreed. A couple of months after moving in together, we got engaged on a weekend away in Paris. Years later we often joked about how he imperceptibly wove the threads of our lives together right under my nose. My head stayed buried in the pages of books or on a pillow catching up on nights of no sleep.

In one of the smaller hospitals I worked in during that time, the nights on call were brutal. Barry often got up early to come in and collect me in the car, throwing my bicycle into the boot and enveloping me in a tight hug. He was a quiet support from the day we met, taking a particular pride in that role. He would often join me on nights out with hospital colleagues, especially in the first few years of our life together. He could chat to anyone. Pauper or king, Barry had a good word for everyone.

At that point in my training, I was rotating through posts in smaller hospitals. Smaller hospitals have the advantage that everyone knows everyone. The nurses know everything there is to know about the hospital; the healthcare assistants, the porters and the admission staff know everything there is to know about the town. As a young doctor, rotating through the post, you lean heavily on the permanent staff to fill in the blanks. Also, small hospitals take all kinds of patients through their doors

I was a very junior and inexperienced anaesthesiologist in one such hospital when I first met Jamie. An essential part of training is learning to move with as much grace and skill as you can muster between different age groups, and to expect a level of complexity and specialty often found in the setting of a small regional hospital. An added element of uncertainty was that this evening on call happened to be 31 October, Halloween.

Jamie was four years old and had been to a party in a neighbour's house. He was dressed in costume as an Egyptian mummy. We met because I was called to help put in a drip for some fluids. Not much information was forthcoming on the phone, except for one of the emergency department nurses' voices in the background: 'Tell her she needs to come down to us now!' I recognised Phil's voice, the voice of experience, as our paths had crossed on quite a few evenings in the four months since I had arrived. I finished what I was doing in the operating room and headed down to see what was going on.

Jamie was sitting bolt upright in a charred mess of bandage material on a trolley, surrounded by noise and the movement of people around him. I looked at him and he looked at me. I experienced what I christened in my mind as the 'halo'. I have felt it many times since then. Perhaps it's just a trick of perception or memory, I don't know.

The halo is the image my mind sees when another human is dying. There is an appearance of a human, yet there is an animal terror that is like a silent drowning. It is in the eyes of a person who can feel how close they are to death. Huge open pupils, their eyelids splinted back. Breath that has begun to slow, sometimes with a whispered grunt at the end of each deliberate indrawing of air. There is a colour in the skin around the edge of the person's lips that accompanies this picture. That colour doesn't have a name, but it is grey and white and purple, all at the same time. Every doctor who works with acutely sick patients knows that hue and respects it.

As I saw Jamie's face, time passed the same as always on the clock, but internally I felt it slow. Deep inside I was terrified too. Everything else in the room disappeared, and communication occurred without words. It was as if a light shone within my mind on the person in trouble, and all around them fell into darkness. There was nothing in the darkness that I needed to see. Every one of my nerve cells fired and transmitted energy in reply to the person in the light. For a split second we shared a primal fear.

There is a halo of urgency and light that tethers me.

Jamie's lips were hugely swollen and pale, as were his gums. I could see his gums easily as his lips were retracted with the swelling. If you had just glanced, you would bizarrely have thought he was smiling. Somewhere behind this frightening picture was a beautiful healthy boy. His cheeks were already starting to blister; his eyelids and fringe were singed. I knew the swelling and blistering were also developing in his airways and lungs. The delicate lining tissues were filling with fluid, spilling over into the magical air sacs.

If left unmanaged, Jamie's airways would close completely, and he would experience precisely what he could feel was coming.

'We need to go to the operating room,' I said. 'Now.'

Although I'd read about this kind of case, I'd never done one before. I called the consultant, and he talked me through the steps to take, making it clear that he had 'full confidence' in me, which meant that he was not coming in from home to do it. Medicine was still extremely hierarchical in those years and even calling the consultant to ask for help was frowned upon. As inexperienced doctors, we managed the medical care of very sick people, many of whom we were too inexperienced to realise how close to death they were.

In the operating theatre, Sinead, the anaesthetics nurse, had laid out every piece of airway equipment she could find. There were instruments in paper packets I had never seen before, never mind knowing what they were meant to be used for.

The surgical registrar came to assist, though he said he didn't think he'd be much use. We stood huddled together fearfully in the silence of the operating room, waiting for the lift doors to open. All this fear we swallowed out of view, as Phil and the porter, Joe, wheeled Jamie in on the trolley, his mother clutching his little hand. For a moment my eyes fell on the paper sheet covering the trolley. There is a horrible indignity to those paper sheets that are used throughout hospitals, although I understand their practicality. Humans who are dying should have soft, clean laundry.

I gently anaesthetised Jamie on his mother's lap, with a mask held to his face, starting slowly with a low dose, gradually building it up. 'Good boy ... You're OK, Jamie,' I murmured over and over to him. When he was deeply sleeping, Phil put her arm around Jamie's mother and walked her out of the room. She turned and looked at her son again through metal guardrails, lying on the hospital trolley. That lingering, loving look hooked deep into my soul.

'Please?' she said to me.

'I will,' I replied.

We were lucky that night. A tiny breathing tube slipped through his vocal cords, and it was just big enough to support his burnt lungs. We phoned both children's intensive-care units in the city and he was accepted to one.

An ambulance crew arrived, and we brought Jamie to where he would be safely cared for. The paediatric intensive-care team chastised us when they saw how tiny the breathing tube was that we had placed into Jamie's lungs. That bugged Sinead, and she grumbled about it on the way back to our own hospital. 'They haven't a bloody clue,' she raged.

I sat back, rested my head against the seat and closed my eyes. I didn't care that the tube wasn't perfect. Or about their harsh words on how we had managed the case. It was enough. We had done enough. Jamie was safe now, and he would recover. Our promise to his mum had been kept. We were able to leave him in safe hands and he was not my responsibility any longer. 'It's better to be lucky than good' is a medical saying that has its roots in experiences like that. I sometimes kick myself for promising parents that we'll do our best. Do they know how limited our powers often are? Would it be more accurate to offer the less generous reassurance that we'll do what we can?

Fast forward to 2025, to our large, busy PICU where we receive hundreds of children from small hospitals each year. As a consultant, I have never forgotten how frightening it is to have the life of a small child in your hands when you feel you lack the skills, experience or equipment to deal with the case. It is terrifying. It is run–out-of-the-room terrifying – but you cannot run. You must stay and try to help.

Critically ill small children and babies do not make up the bulk of the work of small hospitals and it is challenging to maintain every skill gained in training, which may have taken place many years ago. I recognise the fear on the faces of staff when such children arrive and the tremendous relief that rushes through them when they have handed the responsibility to us. 'You're probably pretty happy to hand over this little fella now I'd say?' I'll tease them with humour and share in their glow of release.

The transporting team always walk back down the corridor out of PICU feeling lighter, giddily joking with each other about finding food before getting back on the road. Feedback on their performance can be given with measure and kindness and can wait for another time.

9. Unconditional Love

'The ultimate lesson for all of us is unconditional love,
which includes not only others but ourselves as well.'
Elisabeth Kübler-Ross

I had trained as an anaesthesiologist with adult or mixed adult and child patients for several years so it was time to do a specialty paediatric post. A six-month spell of training with babies and children is a mandatory training experience, even if the anaesthesiologist has no intention of working with children in the future. Most of us dreaded it.

Anaesthesia and critical care for small babies and children has the reputation of being technically challenging, with the added presence of at least one parent. That parent carries their hopes and dreams for their child and scrutinises the body language of every staff member they meet. Just as the lioness lies on the savannah scanning the horizon for danger to her cubs, a human parent is attuned to every change in facial expression, every change in atmosphere in the hospital room.

Within weeks of my having started in the children's hospital, Barry was getting used to me telling him tales about cute little children and the funny things they said. By now we had been engaged for a few years, and we both wanted children in the future.

Children's hospitals are staffed by people committed to fighting hard for each child. The hierarchy between professionals is flatter in paediatric medicine and there is a strong sense of purpose and camaraderie. The combination of parents and staff all striving for the very best is one of the enchanting features of paediatrics. But it also leads to a highly charged environment.

I met April towards the middle of my first paediatric training period. Her story captures the incredible emotional investment by staff that is so frequently encountered. I walked into PICU and saw her in the centre of her tiny room. She was sitting up in a highchair, pointing at what she wanted, like a tiny queen. Tight blonde curls, blue eyes that mirrored the September sky. She had never been outside.

April, darling of the paediatric intensive-care unit.

She was almost two years old when I wandered in looking for my supervising senior doctor. At first glance, anyone would wonder why she was there at all, royally holding everyone in her sway, while she was the captive. Jessica and Shane, her parents, hadn't been able to take her home as there was no community support, like home nursing hours, or medical equipment suitable for parents to use. She had complicated medical problems that needed specialised nursing and equipment. She had lived all her life in the care of the nursing and medical staff, with her parents visiting. She had been born in a nearby maternity hospital and transferred to our care. She had many mammies, the nurses competing to look after her. Over the weeks, which turned into months, she developed and grew plump and demanding. She couldn't talk, but she knew how to make her wishes known to all, with a pout and a shake of her head: 'No, no, NO.'

For the few months I worked there I, too, fell for her little ways. We always spoke about her as if her stay was temporary, 'when April goes home', as if no one wanted to acknowledge how long she'd been with us and how unlikely it was that she'd leave. Some weeks we would be more optimistic, depending on what someone had heard through the hospital grapevine about 'getting April home'.

After a period of intense negotiation and training of staff outside the unit, she finally left PICU and went to the ward. There were pink balloons and cakes to celebrate the huge step of leaving our odd world. It was two weeks shy of April's second birthday. Jessica cried and, in that moment, I could see how even the strangest of worlds becomes safe. It was a square clinical room, the lights perpetually switched on. It was rarely quiet, and it was home.

The PICU nurses held Jessica in a tight hug and told her that everything would be so much better out on the ward, and that in no time she would be home. April and her parents had accumulated so many toys, clothes and books, it took several trips up and down the stairs to move her out of her first home.

Once she was up on the ward, we didn't see April so much, except to pop up and wave at the end of a shift. She and her parents were genuinely missed in PICU. A photograph of her sitting on the lap of Cheryl, one of the Filipina PICU nurses, hung on the wall in the staff tearoom, in the same way that staff shared new-baby pictures. The next goal was to source funding to support her discharge home – for real – to a house that was waiting for the family. It looked like April might go home after all.

But everything changed in a matter of hours. Influenza ripped through the local community that year, a particular strain that became known as swine flu. We hadn't seen serious cases of influenza for years, but toddlers with racking coughs and older children with sky-high temperatures were arriving in droves. A couple of children with influenza infection of their lungs had to be admitted to PICU. The illness was everywhere. Immunisation rates for all common viral infections in childhood had fallen, partly due to the ease that sets in when vaccines are so effective that no one can remember how horrible the sicknesses were, and partly due to fears that vaccines could cause serious problems in previously healthy children.

Still waiting on the ward to go home, April caught influenza. The ward paged me and asked me to review her. When I arrived the atmosphere was tense: I knew that the nursing staff were worried. I went into April's room and was shocked to see her lying lethargic and grunting. Her skin was an angry red, with splashes of dark red and purple. There was hardly any sign of the cute little princess we adored. The small room was warm, but that could not have explained her raised temperature. Her little face was suffused and sweating, her blonde curls now wet and matted. When I put my hand on her chest to examine her further, the heat under my fingertips frightened me. Her heart was racing, an overheating engine under the bonnet of her fragile chest. I spoke to Jessica and explained that April needed to come back to PICU urgently. 'Oh, thank God,' she said, 'thank you,' and she hugged me in relief.

Funding had been sourced to make a mini hospital for her at her home, and her parents had started training to use the medical equipment and give her all her medicines. Influenza knocked off-kilter the delicate balance that had been created for her on the ward. She had weathered so many storms in her life, it was impossibly unfair that this would bring her back to us in PICU, delaying the plans to discharge her.

Initially we thought that this was just a setback. Her further deterioration happened in what felt like minutes but was actually a few horrible hours. April became sicker. We changed her medications, went to the maximum on antibiotics, increased her breathing help and added support for her heart. Through the night, she struggled. We all wrestled with the sense of unreality that this was happening at all. I saw the nurses exchange glances of worry. There was mostly silence in the room as the minutes ticked by. Her nurses, who knew April like the palms of their hands, were aware that we were losing the fight. Staff from the ward where she had been cared for came to see how she was doing and left in tears.

The frantic nature of the first few hours of her admission back into PICU became a slow dwindle without words. I hardly had to say anything to Jessica and Shane, as they were there throughout her slide towards death. She changed from pink to blue, mottled and limp. Her beautiful personality had gone.

April left the body that had kept her chained to intensive care for two years.

Death in a child is a visceral, visual experience. Into the small hours, relatives of Jessica and Shane arrived, and staff appeared in waves from other parts of the hospital. There was nothing to do but stand around. No one ever realises that standing around, murmured words and cups of tea are all that happens after a loved child dies. There's an empty space in the universe that we must stand in, drink tea and hold each other. There, we marked the fact that April had been present in our lives.

The nurses were heartbroken. They knew how to care for each other, cried and hugged. As the early day staff came on duty, they cried too. Everyone had a favourite story to tell about April's indomitable personality and her parents' strength. To say the staff loved her like their own is not enough: she was their child in the way that any child belongs to its whole family.

The next morning a fresh consultant came on duty. 'How was your night?'

'It was terrible,' I said.

'Why?'

'April died.'

'Oh,' he said. Silence. 'April? Our April?' he asked.

'Yes, our April,' I replied.

Silence.

'Right then. Let's start the handover round,' he said, with a false brightness.

As a doctor of several years' experience, I had seen plenty of people die, peacefully and otherwise, but I had never experienced the sudden death of a patient to whom I felt an emotional connection. I didn't know what to do with my feelings and was convinced I had no right to be distraught. April wasn't my child; I had known her only a few months as a junior doctor, passing through on a training rotation. I went home in pieces, thinking there must be something wrong with me.

Later that day I went to my new nephew's christening. I sat in the church pew among his proud family. I was bone-tired and heartsore. Looking at the peachy loveliness of the baby, I cried for all that April wasn't, and for all that we had gone through in the day and night before. Blissfully oblivious of my work, my family smiled knowingly, believing I was broody.

Two days later, I applied for a job at a management-consultancy firm. 'I'm done. I'm leaving medicine,' I told my fiancé. It was a month to our wedding.

I didn't get to the second round of interviews. My training rotation in medicine for children came to an end, and with relief I returned to a post in adult anaesthesiology. I resolved to avoid practising in such a tumultuous specialty ever again.

But life had another plan.

Within a year of our marriage, our first son, Arthur, arrived to unpick my perfectionism and melt my heart. For the first time, as a mother, I felt the same unconditional love I had observed in April's room. Everything changed when I became a mother, especially in my capacity to be a doctor. That is not the case for every doctor, but it was essential in what lay ahead for me. Life, with its powerful swells and crashing waves, would wash me back to medicine for children but would throw me a life-raft: my own family.

10. Vision

Despite my doubts about my medical training, I remained on the programme. I rotated through different training posts, trying to balance long shifts and frequent on-call duties with being a mother to our toddler son. We were fortunate that Barry's job had more regular hours and we fell into a pattern of my leaving for work in the early morning, with him dressing and feeding Arthur and bringing him to crèche. Our days were busy but we were close. Barry had an unwavering belief in our shared capacity to grow our family and succeed in our careers.

The end of my structured training programme was within sight, just a couple of jobs left. Then another doctor swapped post towards the end of the postgraduate training programme, and I was shuffled back to paediatrics. The sliding doors of Fate.

It was during this job I witnessed an interaction that changed my life. Maggie was a six-month-old who been admitted to PICU overnight. She was critically ill with a severe bacterial infection in her bloodstream. She had had many infections over her short life, and we were pursuing investigation of her immune system, as she did not appear to mount any of the expected immune response to sepsis. We were gathered as a group at the end of PICU attending to another new admission when the emergency bell rang from Maggie's room.

Martina was a newly appointed consultant in paediatric intensive-care medicine. She was a forthright woman from the west of Ireland and had the enviable confidence of a well-trained doctor who loved their work. She dashed into Maggie's tiny room as we all piled in with resuscitation equipment. Martina took control and gave everyone tasks to do, including directing me to start compressions on Maggie's little chest. The scene was chaotic, noisy and distressing. Nurses came in and went out of the room, a radiographer appeared to take a chest X-ray, and blood-test bottles were filled in a hurry and dispatched to the laboratory. Throughout this disorder, Martina instructed and led. She seemed to relax a little, in acceptance that this was where we found ourselves right now.

'Maggie's mum is sitting outside,' said the nursing shift leader to Martina. 'What will I do with her?'

'Jesus Christ! She's the baby's mother! Get her in here!' replied Martina, with a conviction I found astounding. This was 2003 and we were not yet at the stage of acknowledging the feelings of our patients' families in such a raw, empathic way.

'Are you sure?' said the nurse. 'It's very upsetting to see all of this.'

'It's a hell of a lot more upsetting not to be with your dying baby,' shot back Martina. 'Maggie is her baby. Her mother should be here.' Those words echoed around the room.

A slight, trembling woman was brought in. Martina took her hand and drew her up to the head of the cot, where Martina was standing and working. 'Put your hand here.' She placed Maggie's mother's hand on the baby's little head. 'Maggie knows you're here now.'

We continued our efforts to revive Maggie and bring her back to a life that would bring joy to her mother, memories for her grandparents and the magical potential that was rightfully hers. We couldn't.

Martina bustled everyone out of the room, except Maggie's mother and me.

I started to leave, but she commanded, 'Stay here,' and I knew by her tone not to disagree. The cot was a mess of blood tubes, drips and gauze squares from blood tests and giving medications in an emergency. She guided Maggie's mum to a chair and then gently lifted Maggie from the shredded, blood-spattered sheets she lay on and placed her in her mother's arms. She removed Maggie's breathing tube. 'There,' she said. 'Now you can see her beautiful face again.' Martina sat down beside them and murmured soft words to the mother. She told her that her baby was dead and would not return to life.

'Tell me, how will I bury my baby?' the mother wailed in response. The room was completely silent, except for her anguished sobs.

I stood in the middle of the shocking mess, bins pushed against the wall, cot at an angle, empty packaging and crumpled bed linen thrown in a pile on the floor. I waited for Martina to tell me what she wanted me to do next. The clock on the wall showed ten past eleven and the hands seemed to stick there, no matter how long I waited.

Martina stood. She beckoned to me to follow her. As we went out of the door, a nurse slipped past us and went into the room. 'You've got to do the right thing. You had to see what it is to do the right thing,' Martina said. 'You must always think about the child. Think about doing the right thing for the child. Nothing else matters.' Then she turned and strode off up the corridor, issuing orders to the various people she passed.

In that hour, I had observed a doctor step into the experience of another human. She had taken me with her, in an act of deliberate guidance. Standing in the shoes of a bereft mother, I absorbed the emotional and intellectual fuel that would propel me in a different direction, as a person and as a doctor.

11. Tennis Shorts

'The cure for broken dreams is to dream again, and deeper.'
C.S. Lewis

Billy was a legendary consultant in the children's hospital where I continued to train. He was an anaesthesiologist and a physician in the true sense: he had broad knowledge and skills, and he cared for everyone, patients and staff. He was also a mediator and a tremendous teacher, who displayed his own vulnerability.

One Sunday afternoon, as registrar on duty, I called Billy. I described Gavin, the two-year-old child I had just assessed in the emergency department. We discussed the issues, the results of the blood tests and the rash that had started to appear across the little boy's feet. One of the challenges that doctors and nurses face when caring for young children is the speed at which their condition can change. It is because all their organs are in peak condition so they make silent compensatory changes to maintain an outward normal appearance. Until there are no compensations left to make and collapse occurs. At this point, Gavin was breathing fast, he had pains in his legs, and he was freezing. We suspected that he most likely had early meningococcal sepsis, although he was sitting up awake and interactive enough to push away anyone who came near him.

We talked about a plan of treatment for Gavin, and I set up my equipment. Billy had suggested I ask one of the senior PICU nurses to come to the emergency department and assist me. Mobile phones were not widely used by consultants at this time – it was mostly long-range pagers – so he gave me a landline number to call him on if I needed help.

I took my time explaining to Gavin's mother, Sheila, what I was going to do and why. She wore an expression I saw many times over the years – a mixture of relief that Gavin was to be treated straight away, and terror for what might happen next. He was sitting on her lap now, whimpering softly into her chest. The PICU shift leader, Jenny, had arrived to help, and I slowly administered the medication that would sedate Gavin to allow us to begin full critical-care support.

I lifted his limp little body off Sheila's lap and a nurse brought her outside. Standing above Gavin, I saw his life and colour leave his body. His heart had stopped beating. The tiniest dose of sedation had unmasked the enormous effort his body had been making to survive the storm of sepsis. His tiny body had been freezing because all his blood pressure had been squeezed into the centre of his body, keeping blood flow to his heart and brain. Sepsis had made his circulation completely inadequate, through a combination of increased tissue demand and a direct toxic effect on his heart.

Jenny and I jumped into our resuscitation steps, ably helped by the rest of the doctors and nurses. Within seconds Billy arrived, though I hadn't had a chance to give his number to anyone. He walked into the department in white tennis clothes, saw what was happening and joined the team. After ten minutes, Gavin's heart began beating again weakly. We continued to support his heart and lungs while assembling our equipment to move him to the PICU. Billy quietly asked me to go out and talk to Sheila, then bring her in to see Gavin. She cried when I described how terribly sick Gavin was, and then she thanked me. At that I felt a rush of shame because he had had a cardiac arrest under my care. Without saying more, I brought her in to see her son.

As quickly as we could, we headed for the lift, pushing Gavin and equipment on a trolley. In the lift, I looked at Billy. 'How did you know to come?' I asked him.

He shrugged. 'I wanted to see his rash with my own eyes ... I must have had a hunch.'

Hours passed in the PICU. Gavin had several briefer cardiac arrests, and it was a battle to stabilise his condition. It was now about 4 a.m. Billy sat at the nurses' station, his head in his hands, his tennis shirt crumpled and stained. Bizarrely I wondered about the game that he had abandoned hours before.

He lifted his head and looked at me. 'How could we have done this better?' he asked. Without waiting for an answer, he shook his head morosely and said, 'We'll have to do better the next time.' Then he stood and handed me a prescription for an antibiotic. 'Get this filled in the hospital pharmacy before you leave after handover. Take it for two days.' I nodded sadly.

It was with relief that I handed over all the PICU patients that morning, including Gavin. The pharmacy gave me the antibiotics I needed to ensure that neither I nor anyone close to me developed meningococcal sepsis. The pharmacist reminded me that, as a side-effect, the medication would turn my bodily fluids orange for a day or so. I popped the first capsule into my mouth as I walked to the bike shed to head for home. It stuck in my oesophagus, a lumpy pain in my chest.

There was a cold dread in my heart when I collected Arthur from crèche later that day. It was a couple of moments' walk from our house, and I had slept fitfully for a few hours before stirring to go and fetch him. I hadn't seen him for almost three days because I had spent forty-eight hours continuously on shift in the hospital. I couldn't wait any longer to snuggle him. My husband had dropped him at the crèche that morning on his way to work, telling the staff that I'd be there after lunch.

Arthur bounced out of the door to the Toddler Room and ran straight into my arms, tiny navy dungarees with a red and navy striped shirt underneath, curly red hair and big smiles. Alive. So alive. I picked him up and held him tight to my body. He wriggled and protested. His mad energy, his hot breath on my face and his feisty giggles shoved images of Gavin's lifeless body in front of my eyes.

We went to the playground on the way home, and I stood behind my little son, pushing him on the baby swing. Filled with despair, fear, guilt and shame. Tears streaked orange down my face, stigmata of the distressing experience, as if normal tears could never be enough to express the depth of my sadness.

A few days later, Billy sought me out in the operating room. We sat together and he asked how I felt after Sunday's events. Straight away, I told him how upset I was. 'I know I didn't do it all right, I'm sorry,' I said.

He sat back in his chair. 'Oh, no, my dear,' he said. 'I want to learn from this. That's what I meant when I said we've got to do better. We must do that with every single patient. Every time. Every day, think about what you did that was good, and think about what you could have done better. That's what I try to do. We must always be learning.' He reached forward and squeezed my hand. 'You're wonderful. You saved Gavin's life,' Billy said. 'You care a lot about what you do. That will keep you right.'

I explained about the anxiety I had for my own child's health, that he would develop meningococcal sepsis or any other of the myriad terrifying illnesses we saw each day. Billy told me he had felt the same fear with his children, especially when they were small. I felt a little better when I knew that a consultant with years of experience under-stood and empathised.

We moved on and discussed the second-by-second events and the steps we had taken on Sunday, and if we were faced again with the exact same situation, how we might improve the details. At the end, we stood up. I felt lighter.

Billy wrapped me in a hug and we laughed.

The lessons I learnt from that week were many. They were medical and they were personal. I saw clearly how my experiences at work would impact on my feelings for my own children. That frightened me and I felt the weight of it on my shoulders as a mother. It seemed to be part of the terms and conditions of being a parent and a doctor to very sick children. That duality would inform my relationship with my husband and my children, even as they grew into adulthood.

Over the years that followed, Barry often commented that it was sometimes difficult to parent with me because I had such an altered sense of achievement, danger and pain. When our little daughter etched pictures onto every surface of our newly renovated home, I thought it was marvellous. I never worried about homework or grades. It was frustrating for Barry, but he would smile and shrug his broad shoulders when I reminded him that they were diamonds, each a unique jewel that we might only briefly hold.

Gavin recovered completely and was discharged after three weeks.

Over the following months I made up my mind to complete my training and go to Melbourne, Australia, to work in paediatric intensive care at the Royal Children's Hospital. Barry would take leave from his job and care for Arthur in Melbourne, while I would work and continue my training. Our plans were set.

Except we discovered that we were to be parents for a second time. We were ecstatic, having tried for a couple of years with no sign of another pregnancy. We decided to stick to the plan.

12. Some People Are Lucky

'Luck is what happens when preparation meets opportunity.'

Seneca

Estella was born six weeks before we moved from Dublin to Melbourne. She was the healthiest baby and did everything as if she had read the textbook on how to be a perfect baby. We were entranced.

Barry now had two small children to care for in a city we didn't know. He wasn't daunted, packing Arthur and Estella into the buggy and heading off each day to explore every gallery, museum, park and coffee shop in Melbourne – of which there are many.

I went to work. There, I expressed breast milk for Estella in the changing room between caring for patients and dashing to emergencies dotted around the vast world-renowned hospital. The injured and sick children I encountered there were the same as in Ireland. Their parents were upset and exhausted in the same way. The PICU staff had the same tenderness for their precious charges. But with our growing family, I became more aware of how tenuous life is. How everything can change in a second. Especially with toddlers.

Toddlers are mischievous. They are hopelessly attracted to climbing, the higher the better. In the accidents that cause serious injury in children, we see a peak in admissions in two age groups: toddlers and teenagers.

My colleagues and I first met Gabriel in the emergency department. The paramedics had called ahead to let us know they were bringing in a critically injured infant. Gabriel had toppled out of a second-floor window. His mother had just nipped into the bathroom when she heard terrified screaming and roaring from people in the street below.

I've gone to hundreds of these calls and the sense of dread as you wait for the ambulance never leaves me. I feel nauseated as I wait, poisoned by dread. What desperate story is about to unfold as I stand in the resuscitation bay, checking equipment, drawing up medications, standing and waiting, waiting for sirens? Hoping there might be a follow-up call to stand down. Maybe exchanging a bit of banter with a colleague you haven't seen in a while. But it's always muted. We fall into silence.

The sirens seemed to start abruptly and within seconds they were there. We got to work. There is a rhythm to how a well-trained resuscitation team works together. We are held by that rhythm and the tasks. In a strange way they allow us not to focus on the beautiful child. That would be too raw and distracting. If we think only of the child and the horror of what they might be feeling, we will be rooted to the spot and incapable of helping them. We hold those thoughts slightly away from us. They can come later.

I hold the small syringes that contain a drug to induce unconsciousness, a strong opiate painkiller, and a drug to stop Gabriel's muscles moving. I have calculated the doses based on a weight I have estimated for him. I repeat the calculations and check the ampoules from which I have drawn the drugs. Once I administer them into his veins, a line will be crossed from which we cannot step back. Those medications will rest his brain and body and allow us to support him using equipment and machines. But they are also potent drugs with frightening side-effects that must be anticipated and managed in a broken body. And we don't yet know how damaged Gabriel is.

Gabriel's mother, Maria, was brought into the resuscitation room to be with him before we took him to the radiology department for scans. Her face crumpled into tears and she sobbed, shouting his name over and over again. Eventually she sat in a chair beside him, continuing to whisper his name. We explained what we were going to do next, what might happen, what we were worried about. Looking into her eyes, I could see she wasn't taking in any of this. It's so often the case. Then it becomes the way in which the words are said, a warm squeeze of a hand that might linger. The trust of a stranger is humbling, as she quietly handed over her child to people she had never met before. With my rational brain I knew she had no choice, but it still impressed me that Maria believed we would care for Gabriel. She knew nothing about us, not even our names, never mind our qualifications, yet she trusted us. We were bound by this trust. In effect, there was an unspoken promise. We promise to serve.

Later in the PICU, we listed Gabriel's injuries as we handed over his care from one shift to another. It was a mesmerising and scary collection. He had sustained damage from the top of his head to the soles of his feet, but somehow he was stable. He was asleep under the heavy influence of medication, and he had tubes and infusion lines coming from many parts of his little body. We gave him a blood transfusion, a red gift of service from another stranger. We told Maria we must wait. We don't find waiting easy ourselves. Our natural inclination and training mean that we like doing things. If we do things, people will get better. Doing things feels like progress. Patience and time can be friends to the treatment and support that have been put in place. But waiting is taxing on everyone's nerves. Over the days of waiting, Maria told the nurses about her life, her baby Gabriel and the hopes and plans she had for him.

Maria brought in photographs of Gabriel and his father, who lived in another country at that moment but was trying to get to Melbourne. Our social worker was busy supporting the little family. Visas and flights entered the conversation, and whether there was time to organise everything before Gabriel . . . died. No one wanted to say that word but, of course, we must say it aloud.

We had a brain-activity monitor on Gabriel's head. It showed that his brain was having seizures. We treated them with drugs to reduce the metabolic rate of his brain and to calm the electrical storms that were taking place in its cells. It added to the strain in the room. We waited some more.

My colleague, more experienced than I, came in to look at the brain monitor. 'It looks OK,' she said. 'I think this little boy will be OK.'

Maria heard her say those magical words and cried. I caught a sob in my throat and bit my lip. I saw the PICU nurse doing the same.

Several weeks later Gabriel, now healed and intact, was in Maria's arms, waving bye-bye to everyone.

Why did he live and another child might not? We will interrogate the details later, searching for clues and ways to improve.

Maria smiled, clutching him tightly to her, and that was enough.

Some people are lucky, and that seems to be part of the essence of existence. Seeing the fleeting nature of fortune colours how we live. At the end of each shift, I felt so grateful to go home and bury my face in the warm smell of our two little children. Their presence in my life gave me unending sustenance. To them, I was their mother. I was safety, nourishment, warmth, guidance and unconditional love. They gave that back to me a thousand-fold.

13. Trusting a Stranger

'We are each of us angels with only one wing, and we can only fly by embracing one another.'

Luciano De Crescenzo

'I trust you to look after my little girl,' said Fiona's mother, Sarah.

The trust that parents place in us is profound, but it's unusual to hear those words of affirmation spoken. The creation of trust can happen very quickly, and I'm often amazed that, when the situation is critical, people reach for trust and hand over their child to strangers. Trust is an essential ingredient of how we work together. When it's lost because something has happened and people feel let down, it is incredibly difficult to regain. This prompts a cycle of fear, questions, scrutiny of all detail and a continuing sense for families that medical care is not being delivered to the highest standard, or that staff don't care enough about their child.

Fiona was five years old and had a complicated cancer that needed many rounds of chemotherapy, several intensive-care admissions and a bone-marrow transplant. Now her body was rejecting the new cells. It was a grave situation, and the outlook was bleak.

'Do you think it's hopeless?' Sarah asked.

'No. We'll tell you when we think it's time for us to stop,' I replied.

'OK. I've decided to trust you,' she said again. She was a forthright Australian woman, but there was something about the way she said this that made me wonder what had occurred before Fiona was admitted to PICU.

Sarah sat by Fiona's bed with a photograph of the two of them on her lap. She watched us work on her daughter. I asked her about the photo. In it, Fiona was a flower girl at Sarah's sister's wedding. She and Sarah glow with colour, health and love for each other. It had been taken the summer before Fiona's illness had been diagnosed. They were insep-arable, Sarah said. Fiona's father had a new family, so it was just the two of them.

The hours ticked by. One of the shift leaders joined the bedside nurse to help with medication preparation. Then she sat down beside Sarah and kept her company in silence. The PICU nurses are naturally intuitive, and many can sit and hold a parent without speaking, trying to fix emotions or making promises.

We were in the endless period of waiting for treatment to work. Waiting for the human body to decide if this time it will release white cells from the marrow. If this time the medicines will be accepted into the arms of their receptors and the sickened cells will recover. This is what I picture during these hours. If the treatment does not appear to work, we will go back to the start of what we know and try another path. Until we simply run out of paths to try.

Few people outside medicine understand how vast parts of our body are like the bottom of the ocean: we can never see these parts; they will only tease us with clues. Investigations, radiological scans, blood levels are all clues. Added to the secrets that the body and brain keep is the mysterious interaction between chemicals – medications – and the body.

Drugs are developed stringently through grades of exposure in laboratories, animals and human testing. Their indications and doses are modified, and their side-effects are categorised and published. Yet there remains an unquantifiable interaction in each individual human. All of us have the mundane experience where one antibiotic upsets our stomach, but our brother can take it with no problem. Or one person thrives for years on a combination of drugs to control their blood pressure, and another develops side-effect after side-effect. Is it luck or genetics, or is it where our limited state of knowledge has us right now? It's probably a bit of all three.

After years of learning rules and numbers to describe the human body, I am left in awe of the contradiction that exists in our individuality.

Over the week of Fiona's stay in PICU her condition stabilised and then improved. The improvement, when it came, arrived quickly. Fiona woke up, wanted all equipment removed and asked for her nappy to be taken away. 'I want apple juice!' she said, as her breathing tube came out. A few days later she bounced out of PICU, full of little-girl chat and cuddles for her mother.

Sarah was overjoyed and tearful with gratitude. 'I thought I had nothing left,' she said. 'I thought all our chances were gone . . . but you gave us another shot.'

By now, Sarah had us all in tears with her, as she spoke of her total desolation just a week or so earlier. We finally allowed ourselves to see how close Sarah had come to losing the most precious thing of all.

What made the difference for Fiona? We don't know. After her, there may be Sadhbh, Poppy, Finian . . . Some will recover but others will not. Balancing the delicate nature of trust with the duty to communicate how uncertain the outcome is from any critical illness is very demanding.

It is overwhelming to ask relatively unknown people, who are terrified their child is going to die, to trust you, and at the same time to understand that you cannot promise their child will survive.

I have got the subtlety of this message wrong on occasion.

Once, the parents of a child asked that their child be brought to another hospital as they could not trust me: I had told them we were unsure what the problem with their child's heart was but would do our best to find out. Embarking on a conversation of such a delicate nature would be challenging if you knew the people you were sharing the information with. Doing so when you are strangers to each other is another hurdle entirely. I was blessed to be part of a supportive team who pulled around and healed the rift.

Trust is won on the basis that all that has gone before has shown that someone or some service is trustworthy.

When we admit a patient from another hospital or service where a family believes the best care has not been given, it's even more difficult and important to establish an open dialogue and try to grow a tiny flicker of trust into a more enduring flame. Fiona had initially come in through another hospital, when she was feeling sick, but the signs were not easy to see. Sarah felt she wasn't listened to and that there had been a delay in starting treatment. If her concerns had been investigated earlier, would Fiona have avoided a life-threatening complication and illness?

Sarah always had the right idea about trust. She called it out. She was able to show her upset and disappointment that some aspects of care were not what her daughter needed at the time. Like many people she bottled her despair to tolerate the agony of uncertainty, and she saw that in each moment there were good things to focus on. She achieved an immense act of courage – she opened her heart and allowed herself to grow to trust us, and this was not only because Fiona came back.

14. We Are So Sorry

'In each loss there is a gain, as in every gain there is a loss, and with each ending comes a new beginning.'
                                                            Buddhist proverb

Throughout our training to work with patients, we place a lot of emphasis on the acquisition of knowledge. As I spent more time in intensive care in Melbourne, I began to see how the tiniest part of knowledge is facts. Knowledge requires understanding and a well of empathy to draw on as that knowledge is shared.

All babies are beautiful, and every now and then a baby is so beautiful that it is beyond comparison. That special baby is your own little one. However, one soft, perfectly pink baby who was not my own never leaves my mind: Sophie. She was the perfect weight and had been born easily, without a hair on her head touching anything except the gentle guiding hand of her midwife. She gurgled and cooed after feeding and slept with her arms thrown above her head, in the complete innocence of the newborn. She did not appear sick.

She was not sick yet.

Sophie and her mother came over to PICU from the maternity unit to see if anything could be done. She was fifteen hours old. Although it had been explained with kindness by the most senior doctors at several outpatient visits during late pregnancy that Sophie would not survive more than a week or so after her birth, her mother quietly asked if we could make an exception and bring her to PICU to meet the specialists. The same specialists who said they could not offer Sophie anything. Her mother wanted to know what they knew and hear it again.

The cardiologist on duty that weekend shrugged his shoulders apologetically as he came over to PICU for a chat and to make the referral. 'We have been through all the information several times at our joint conference, and the baby's parents know all of that, but . . .' he said. He was asking us to allocate Sophie a bed. We do not work in PICU to have hearts of stone and turn away from need. We staffed a bed and accepted her care.

We repeated some of the tests. We looked together at the images produced by the tests and the measurements. There was no treatment, drug or surgery that would work. Most experienced doctors have worked in big, busy hospitals around the world as part of their training, and we have a network of colleagues internationally with whom information can be shared to double-check that no specialist in another centre could do something. We sent out the measurements for another opinion.

Could you take this beautiful baby and do surgery on her body, knowing that it would fail? Knowing that she would experience pain, but it would not change anything? Knowledge of a condition, how it will progress and steal life, feels like a burden sometimes. Would it be easier on everyone if we knew nothing and Sophie declined at home without reason, then left her parents bereft and unknowing?

We came back into their room and shared our experience, the possible choices, the second and third opinions and all the hard facts with Sophie's parents. 'We are so sorry.'

We waited for them to let us know what their wishes were.

'Thank you for seeing her,' they said. 'We just needed to know for sure, although we knew it ourselves deep down. We'll go back now.'

With a dignity and power no one could ever imagine, Sophie's parents took her back to the maternity hospital, and from there, they went home. At home, after a day or so, Sophie slipped away in their arms, as gently as the breath she had been born with.

It was during my time in Melbourne that I stopped sharing with my husband the human tragedies I witnessed. Barry was immersed in the care of our small children. It was a responsibility he took enormously seriously and his bond with them grew stronger each day. Every tale of loss from the intensive-care unit tore him apart for days.

Not unlike my own father, Barry found it desperately upsetting to know that not every little child went home healthy, with loving parents. During those years I spoke about my experiences less and less. We were a fragile, newly grown family, a kernel of the wider family we had left thousands of kilometres away. We didn't have friends for the first few months and clung to each other. People we met were kind, but we had little support if we needed any. We pushed that thought to the backs of our minds. Exploring Australia and making the most of our time there was a positive focus instead. We became very inventive in packing up four-year-old Arthur and baby Estella and jumping on long-distance coaches, boats and bicycles.

We knew that we would not stay long in Australia, as Barry had put his own career on hold so that we could travel together. We had just less than a year to enjoy a wonderful adventure, our emerging family strength against the world.

15. Giving Is a Choice

'Life's persistent and most urgent question is, "What are you doing for others?"'

Martin Luther King Jr

Making the decision to come back to Ireland was easy. I loved the work in Australia, but Dublin was where our families were. As Arthur and Estella grew, we wanted to be near our parents and siblings so that our children would grow up knowing them. I took a consultant post in anaesthesiology in a large teaching hospital and Barry returned to working in finance.

Our lives were busy, especially when our third child, Dorothea, arrived two years after Estella. She was born a few weeks early and had to stay in the neonatal intensive-care unit until she had gained a bit of weight. We were in the middle of renovating an old house. I attempted to emotionally blackmail the builders into hurrying up and finishing by sticking out my swollen stomach every time I saw them. Later I showed them Polaroids of our baby in the NICU. They said she was lovely and continued to argue about supporting walls and plumbing.

Dorothea grew quickly and came home, the house got finished and I went back to my job when she was six months old. She joined Estella in the crèche down the road from where we lived. Fortunately she settled in easily. Having two young children in childcare and one in primary school was tricky as Barry and I balanced family and work. We always felt as if we were a hair's breadth from everything collapsing on top of us. My youngest sister Louise was an enormous help to us during those frantic family years as she hadn't yet had her own children. Both of our families supported us hugely, and it made returning from Australia entirely justified.

I loved working in the operating room, with a wonderful team and super colleagues, but I missed intensive care. If we had a very sick child in the operating room or on the wards, we transferred their care to the nearest PICU, which was about six kilometres away, as there was no PICU in the hospital where I now worked. Although content in knowing that the child would be well cared for there, I yearned to be with them.

One afternoon I was called to the emergency department to assist with the resuscitation of a teenager. His name was Jack. His story broke everyone's heart. His mother, Patsy, described how he had packed his bag for a football game that was to happen straight after school. He was 'fit as a fiddle' and adored sport. Jack took a big lunchbox that morning as he headed off to school on the bus. He was always hungry.

We got a phone call in the early afternoon about Jack and what had happened to him. My phone rang in my pocket as I stood in the operating room. It was a bit noisy in there so I moved into the back corridor where I could hear the voice of the stressed doctor making the call. I rested my elbows on the window ledge and listened carefully. It was a cold clear day in winter, and I could see the pink sliver of light low in the sky that whispered snow.

Perhaps surprisingly the awful event had occurred in the schoolyard, not on the football pitch. Jack hadn't made it to the pitch. There were several versions of what had happened when Jack and his friends went out for lunch break. Ultimately, after a bit of a kickabout with a ball, Jack had collapsed without warning. His friends and teachers carried out basic life support with chest compressions. They had learnt how to do resuscitation just a few months ago as part of physical education.

As it was a rural school, it took quite a long time for an ambulance to arrive at the scene. First responders for the local area attended and joined the fight to bring Jack back. After more than an hour of attempts to revive him, now in the emergency department, Jack's heart began to beat. In the hour that followed, he had two further cardiac arrests. I discussed his precarious condition with the emergency medicine consultant. 'Is it worth continuing?' he asked.

'Yes, I think so,' I replied. 'We can still make a difference.'

We managed to stabilise his condition a little, and I brought him by ambulance to the PICU in the nearest children's hospital, where I had worked for several years before.

After handing over his care to the PICU consultant who was coming on for the evening, I left. We had acknowledged to each other that Jack was very unlikely to survive such a prolonged cardiac arrest. We told each other stories of children who had made it against the odds, before glumly coming back to the fact that it was almost impossible. Then we talked about the value of PICU admission, even when death was inevitable. 'At least it means that his family will see him again and hold him while he is warm and alive, even if it's just for a day or so,' my colleague said. 'That's got to be worth something. That's valuable.'

In PICU there are a greater number of teenage patients than most imagine. The mixture of tiny babies with illnesses that are often related to their growth and development, and adolescents who present with a completely different profile of disease, means that working in PICU is always engaging and demanding. We walk alongside families and share their stories briefly before our paths diverge again.

I spent the following few days visiting PICU to spend time with my former colleagues and to follow up with Jack. It quickly became clear what would unfold for Jack and his family. I sat with his parents, Patsy and Lar, early on the first morning after his collapse. We discussed the most likely outcome of brain damage or brain death due to injury from lack of oxygen and blood supply during the time that his heart had not been beating. We were joined by a cardiologist who was trying to piece together information to explain why Jack had collapsed.

From the events and pattern of electrical activity that we observed from Jack's heartbeat, it appeared that he had a rare condition that made it more likely for his heart suddenly to stop conducting the electrical signal to tell the heart muscle to squeeze and relax. This condition had been present all of Jack's life, lying silently, a thief in the night. It was most likely genetic in origin.

As the cardiologist said the word 'genetic', I saw terror pass over Patsy's face. She stared at us. Then she said, 'Jesus, the kids.' I knew she was immediately fearing that their other children might be affected. Jack's father pressed on with questions about how Jack's brothers and sisters might be at risk. We explained the assessments that would follow as soon as possible for all their family. The cardiac clinical nurse specialist nodded as she listened, reassured them and made notes to ensure everything was done as we promised.

Late in the afternoon, Jack's brain began to swell in response to the severe injury it had sustained. By morning, it had swollen so much that it had cut off its own blood supply. We again sat with Patsy and Lar. It was so difficult to take this family's hopes and change their lives for ever with our words. Jack lay in his PICU bed, dressed in his club jersey, freckles on his face, a trace of mud still under his nails. He was a beautiful boy who had left home to go to school and play football. It was incomprehensible.

'What happens now?' asked Lar.

That is a question parents often ask when they understand the devastating information we have given them. It is an important question, which shows a shift in the world they have lived in up until now.

Before I could answer, Patsy said, 'Can we donate something?' She faltered. I looked at her but stayed quiet. She took a deep breath and continued, 'Jack's kidneys, his lungs ... can we donate these?'

'Would you like us to see if that is a possibility for Jack?' I asked. 'Your generosity in this most horrible time is incredible. I think that it is possible if that is what you want.' I looked across at Lar. He nodded without speaking.

'If it helps some other poor child, some other family ...' Patsy said in a rush, then put her head into her hands and sobbed. They wrapped themselves around each other, the man and the woman who had grown a wonderful son, now torn up with sorrow.

Jack's sister suggested that some of his friends who had helped look after him in the schoolyard might like to visit Jack and say goodbye. We talked about how we could make it happen, and how it might impact on them. We were anxious that the experience would be overwhelming for those young people, but Patsy was adamant once she got hold of the idea. 'We've got to share Jack with his friends,' she said. 'They need to understand they did good when they were helping him in the yard.'

Two teachers from Jack's school drove up to the hospital with a group of his friends. They waited outside in a room we set aside for them, each wearing the team jersey as they filed in quietly to say goodbye to their friend and teammate. Patsy drew on a strength that was extraordinary to see. She told the boys they had saved Jack's life so that he could help other people, that that was exactly what Jack would have wanted them to do. 'He was a great man for doing things,' she said, 'and him donating his organs is just the kind of fella he is,' she took a slow breath, 'and ye all have helped him do it.'

Father John, our pastoral caregiver, came and said prayers with the boys as they stood awkwardly ranged around Jack's bed. There was a moment of laughter as one of the boys asked about lighting candles, and the PICU nurse explained what oxygen might do with a candle. The humour broke the uneasy spell, and they left the room looking less anxious than earlier.

I thought Patsy was alone with Jack and went back in to see her, to explain the steps that would occur next. I paused at the door as at the back of the room Patsy held a young woman in a hug. The teacher had remained with Patsy and Jack, almost incapable of leaving. Her whole body shook with emotion as she cried. Patsy comforted her, patting her on the back, saying, 'I know, love, I know.'

Discreetly, Jack's nurse and I left them alone.

After multiple tests and much preparation, a big team was assembled to carry out the wishes of Jack's parents. Three days after his collapse, and after his brain had died, Jack donated his organs with the noble intention that they would be given to improve and prolong the lives of other people. His family shared the meaning of giving with everyone.

Jack was wheeled over to the operating room, his bed decorated with county flags, medals he had won and photos of his family. Patsy and Lar walked beside him, dignified and so proud of their son and his siblings.

The family attended the cardiology outpatient clinics in the months after Jack's death for investigation and treatment of his siblings.

They never felt ready to visit the PICU again.

Jack and other sick children quietly gnawed at my core. I recognised that feeling from years ago with Mrs Johnson. Our family were thriving. Our life was comfortable and privileged, and my work was fulfilling. Ambition is commonly understood as rising to the top of some imaginary ladder of success. I wasn't sure that the aim of life was to be satisfied.

In moments of contemplation after long days in the operating room as an anaesthesiologist, I hungered for the chance to invent my own life's meaning and to leave nothing on the table of regrets. I had trained to care for the sickest children, to respond to the pull of a child who needed help. I missed that emotional loop of tug and respond, a need that had been forged when I was a child, watching my sister struggle to breathe.

Around that time, my dissatisfaction was heavily influenced by the philosopher Hannah Arendt who directs us to shift from contemplation to action. She acknowledges the value of thought but challenges the reader to use it to propel them to act. I felt challenged to act with humble purpose, to grow further into the broad role of physician where I became the words I spoke and the actions I took. Inspirational teachers throughout my life had shown the way. It was not meant to be an easy life.

Physician as healer, guide, teacher and advocate.

16. Something That Endures

'When we are no longer able to change a situation, we are challenged to change ourselves.'

Viktor E. Frankl

The discovery that we were having a fourth baby came as a complete surprise to my husband Barry and me. I was now thirty-nine, we had three children and were caught up in the day-to-day of bringing them up. Both of us were working, Barry often travelling with his job and my on-call duties added to the mix. I had been working as a consultant in anaesthesiology for the past seven years, predominantly caring for children, in a large general hospital.

Although I had always wanted to use my training to work in paediatric intensive care, I had made a choice in my career path, a compromise to get my family and husband settled in one place. I had chosen to interview for a general post as an anaesthesiologist in a big teaching hospital. There was no PICU in that hospital, but I felt very lucky and grateful to be successful at interview and to work there. It meant that we could settle down and bring up our children close to both of our families. Women in medicine and many other professions often make such choices along the way, placing family and stability first. Family is the foundation of everything.

At first, I was in denial that I was pregnant, but when the nausea and fatigue, so familiar to me, returned with a vengeance, I couldn't ignore it any longer. One cold Sunday afternoon in March we were in the playground, and I felt so dizzy I had to lie down on a park bench and close my eyes. A concerned woman asked if I was OK. 'I think I'm pregnant,' I said to her.

At last, I'd said the words aloud, to a bemused total stranger, and with it came a rush of anxiety. Our youngest child was four years old. I had long ago given away all the baby stuff. We had decided that our family was complete.

A test confirmed what I already knew. Unlike my previous pregnancies, where I'd waited in hopeful anticipation for the two blue lines to appear, this time I'd hardly had a chance to flush the loo when they were there, as if they had been drawn in crayon by our younger daughter. And there was none of the swooping delight of the previous times. I was in shock. This was not part of the plan.

When the pregnancy was confirmed with an ultrasound scan, I cried at the sight of the tiny mound of cells in my uterus. The midwife smiled and said, 'It's wonderful.'

I said, 'No, it's not. I didn't want to be pregnant.'

Her face fell and she replied, 'There are so many women who want to be in your position right now.' Desperately unhappy and ashamed of how ungrateful I felt, I knew it was pointless to say anything more.

When I was twenty-three weeks pregnant, we went to France on holidays. By now we had become used to the reality of our expanding family, and Barry and I were quietly excited about the little girl who was growing steadily inside me. Each visit to the obstetrician and sonographer only served to deepen the love and anticipation further. Those weeks of pregnancy between five and seven months can be very lovely, if you're lucky.

The children were very excited about the holiday and packed the usual mad collection of toys, swim gear and books. I managed to squash in a few T-shirts and pairs of shorts. They were only the slightest bit aware that another baby was on the way.

After a couple of days in France I began to feel unwell. The fever and fatigue I felt I had put down to the hot weather. I tried to rest. Anyone with small children will know how impossible that is. One baking hot evening as I tidied up after dinner and Barry played cards with the children, I had a horrible sense of dread. A sick, sweaty dread that made tears roll down my face. Barry came over and we hugged. 'What's wrong?' he asked.

'I don't know, I just don't feel good.' I tried to hide my tears from the kids, who were anxiously staring at us from the table. Children are exquisitely tuned in to the feelings of their parents, and I should have known they would not be fooled by the crooked smile I gave them. 'I'm not well so I'm going to bed,' I said, with lots of false reassurance in my voice. 'Nighty night, I love you.'

I woke shaking with sweat and in terrible pain. It was before 5 a.m. and dark. I shook Barry awake. 'I'm in labour,' I said. 'The baby's coming.'

'What?' he asked, dazed with sleep and shock. We woke and dressed the children in our little holiday apartment and went out onto the street, trying to hail a taxi. The pains in my lower belly were getting worse and I had to stop walking each time they came. The children crowded around me each time, upset because I was in pain and scared because I couldn't catch my breath to talk to them. Miraculously, a fire truck passed by. Barry stood in the middle of the road and frantically waved it over. The guys on the truck took one look at me and knew what was going on. They bundled all of us into the back and raced us to the nearest emergency department. The children loved the fire truck and suddenly this new twist in the early-morning scare became a brilliant adventure.

I was assessed in the emergency department by a woman doctor in pink scrubs. When I told her my due date, I heard her say to the nurse behind her that I was twenty-five weeks pregnant. In prematurity outcomes there is a huge difference between twenty-three and twenty-five weeks of pregnancy. Through the my fog of pain, fever and fear, I knew they had calculated backwards, using the French method of measuring the length of pregnancy. I desperately wanted to give my baby the chance that being twenty-five weeks would bring her. I stayed silent. My love for her obscured my usual clarity, like clouds diffusing moonlight.

The doctor found it difficult to place an intravenous drip in my arm because I was shivering, cold and sick by now.

She started me on fluids and a medicine to try to stop labour. I heard her speaking on the phone to another hospital. The one where we had landed was a local injury unit mostly and couldn't care for a mother and baby in premature labour. Outside the door, I could hear our children laughing and chatting to Barry. I put my head back on the pillow, numb with terror. I didn't know what would happen next, but I felt that our family, as we knew it then, was in terrible danger.

Alone this time, I made the next trip by ambulance to Nice. The pains were still coming but they were duller and more widely spaced apart. The doctor came with me, and each time I had a pain, she shook her head crossly, as if it was irritating her.

In Nice, there was calm. The obstetrician assessed me and told me we would be going straight to the operating room for a Caesarean section. She was joined by a male doctor who had a wonderful presence, Dr Amolle. He was a neonatologist, a man in his fifties with an air of kindness and competence. He spoke honestly: 'Your baby is too young and too small.'

'I know,' I said sadly.

'We will try, hmm?' He shrugged his shoulders in the magnificent Gallic way that French men have. 'But here,' and he waved his hand at what I'm not sure, maybe France in general, 'we don't try for life at any cost.' He looked into my eyes as he said this.

'Do you understand me when I say this?' he asked. 'It cannot be life at *any* cost. It's not a good life for you, and it's too much for the baby. It's not a good life for the child.'

He shrugged again. Then he reached out, took my hand in his and squeezed it.

Although there was no decision to be made about my baby's future at that point, I could see that the neonatologist was openly introducing the possibility that there might be a decision for us to make in the future, either later that day or the next. The question about what constitutes a 'good life' is a thorny one. His having brought it into our conversation meant that over the following days we were able to ponder it a little more. No one wants a 'bad life' for their child, but is a bad life the opposite to a good life? And what does a good life look like to our family? These questions had blurry edges to them as they overlapped with many other aspects of our lives, including the potential impact on our other children. The answers to questions about quality or quantity of life are far from being black and white.

Beatrice was delivered by Caesarean section. I heard one tiny cry. I think I heard one tiny cry. I question this with my rational brain and believe it with my sensing heart. She was taken away quickly by the neonatal team. Many hours passed when I did not know if she was alive. I found the language and cultural differences painful and isolating. Left alone in a hospital room, I didn't know where my baby was, who was caring for her or what would happen next. As a doctor, I knew the facts and the likely possible events. As a mother, I felt as if my heart had been torn out and carried away with her body.

That evening Barry was able to visit with the children.

My two little daughters, who were now four and seven years old, had made pictures of the sea, with lots of coloured fish. Barry hung them above my bed. They still talk about those pictures and how they had spelt out 'Happy Birthday' in crayon below the fish, as Beatrice was born the day before my fortieth birthday. But my eldest child, Arthur, who was eleven at the time, stayed silent. He was frozen with fear. He could see how sick I looked, and he knew this family summer holiday had become a nightmare from which we would not awake easily.

I was weak with infection from prolonged rupture of the membranes around Beatrice and was being nursed by complete strangers in a language that was not my own. But the care I received from the nurses transcended words. Sometimes it was hurried and a bit brusque, but mostly it was done with kindness and had a frank, timelessly maternal quality to it.

On one of those first few days, a nurse bathed me in bed. It was one of the most humbling experiences I had ever had. She soaped and washed my body, with a firmness and care, singing what sounded like a nursery rhyme or a lullaby in French as she did her task. I felt completely held. A second nurse joined her, and they towelled my body dry while murmuring softly to each other. I was a little child in their hands, vulnerable and anxious. My own new tiny Beatrice was struggling for life in the NICU, and the nurses did all they could to help me recover so that I could be with her. I had a single Polaroid of her face, which I caressed over and over. These seem like tiny details now, yet they stand out as being sweet and important.

The first day I got out of bed after five days of complete rest, the nurse helping me insisted on calling Barry to tell him that I was 'on the move again'. She encouraged me in every step I took each morning, and she also made a point of checking with the NICU each shift to see if there was any news of Beatrice. My baby was alive and positive messages were relayed back. I had not yet held her or touched her precious face.

I vaguely recall a male medical student sitting beside me at one point and asking me some questions about my medical history and almost feeling as if I was watching myself from across the room. I was incapable of being coherent in his language or in my thoughts, which swam around in their own sea of hope and fear. It all felt surreal, as if I had been anaesthetised and dropped into another world, and I knew I had to try to find my way home.

The days after Beatrice's delivery were mostly a blur. It is extraordinary how quickly time becomes almost irrelevant to you when you are a patient. It seems as if the day has no discernible shape to it, except for the punctuation provided by the nurse coming to administer intravenous antibiotics. It is also extraordinary how important words can be during this disorienting period. A young obstetrician I had not met before came in to check my observations one morning and spoke in English to me. 'Why did you come to France when you were pregnant?' she asked, with a quizzical expression. Before I could put a reply together in my fuzzy brain, she grimaced and continued, 'It was a very stupid idea.' She turned away and left the room. The judgement and the disdain with which she had spoken brought me very low. I had already imagined that Beatrice's early arrival was my fault, and now that doctor had confirmed it.

Beatrice was a beautiful and tiny girl. When I was recovered enough from the significant infection I had at the time of her birth, Barry took me in a wheelchair to the NICU. I adored her from the second I saw her. My heart opened like an empty vessel and flooded with love for her. There is always more love and more space for a child. How could I have doubted that I would not have time and love for her? She had red downy hair above her perfect ears, and long fingers and toes. Her feet were extraordinarily lovely. She slept on her back, a ventilator helping her breathe. We hung some of the girls' pictures on the wall around the incubator.

We decided to take the children home to Dublin as school was starting back after the summer. This was a difficult decision as I did not want to leave my daughter but our other children needed attention, having gone through the experience of their mother suddenly disappearing into hospital while we were on holidays. With huge misgivings, I made the choice to go – but vowed to return as soon as I could get onto a flight back.

The day before Barry and I took the children home to Dublin, they were able to sneak in to see Beatrice briefly. They were thrilled to be allowed in, and we took photographs of each of them holding her hand. My son did not want to: he reached for mine instead and held it long and tight.

I felt broken on the flight home, arms empty, my breasts aching with milk for our baby who had stayed in France.

We were surrounded by tanned holidaymakers, giddy with sunshine and relaxation.

Everything seemed quite hopeful, and we talked a lot about 'when Beatrice comes home'. She was more than a week old, and the shock of her birth had softened. After a day at home in Dublin, settling the children into a semblance of normality, Barry and I tried to figure out a way to take care of everyone. We decided that I would return to France on my own to be with Beatrice, and he would stay with the children in Ireland. Just nine days after serious sepsis and surgery, I dragged breast pump, bags and my own fractured body and soul back to Nice. I knew I was lucky to be able to do that. When a mother's child is sick, we do things that make little sense to the head, yet every good sense to the heart.

There were a few days when all was well with Beatrice, and by extension all was well with us. As a parent your mental health is entirely plugged in to how your child is doing. If they are up, you are up. Quickly the routine began of expressing milk, ringing the bell outside the NICU, sitting beside Beatrice's incubator and then waiting until it was time to do it again, three times a day. I walked outside in a loop around the hospital, soaking up warm sunlight and planning the weeks and months ahead. I was keen to bring Beatrice back to a NICU in Ireland so that we could be together as a family again. But the most important aspect of that plan that we had no control over was when Beatrice would be strong enough. It was difficult to be patient and live in each single, precious day she gave us.

The nurses caring for her were exquisitely gentle. Their fingers and hands fluttered above her body as they worked, and I thought it is truly a gift to nurse a premature infant. They laughed when I thanked them and encouraged me to do her cares, gentle acts of love, tiny morsels of parenting that I clung to – dabbing at her mouth, washing her face and changing her nappy.

Every morning when I walked into the NICU I handed the tiny bottles of expressed milk to Beatrice's nurse. One day the nurse said to me, with irritation in her voice, 'Why do you give these to me?' I said it was milk for Beatrice. She threw her eyes to Heaven and said, 'She is not ready for milk!' I replied that I thought the milk would be stored in the freezer for when she was ready to feed. 'No, we throw it out, so don't bring it again,' she said firmly. That short exchange of words shredded me completely. I continued to express milk to keep up my body's supply, but I didn't bring it into the NICU anymore.

Then came the worrying news that the doctors wanted to talk to me. A different neonatologist from the man I had met on Beatrice's birthday took me through an explanation about a blood vessel that was open between her lungs and heart, and which they felt was stopping her coming off the ventilator. He used the word 'push' several times, to convey that he and the team believed that Beatrice needed a 'push' to make progress. I told him I was a doctor working with children, and he smiled. 'Then you understand.'

I did understand, but I was scared at the idea of my daughter having surgery, especially when everything seemed quite stable. Barry and I talked on the phone about it. We trusted their care and advice and decided to agree to the recommendation to have a surgical closure of the vessel.

It was done the next day. The anaesthesiologist came early in the morning, and we chatted about the plan. I signed the consent form, which was in French. Beatrice was wheeled out of the darkened room she shared with two other babies. As I stood watching her leave, I noticed one of the babies was awake and had now come off their ventilator. Tears of sadness and hope welled in my eyes at the sight of another baby of which I knew nothing. Would my baby do the same? There was a black sliver of envy, too, as I wished and willed my child into that same leap forward. The nurse standing with me must have guessed at the maelstrom of feelings and thoughts I was having: she put her arm around my shoulders and simply said, 'Each baby is different, Madame.'

My beautiful tiny girl returned from surgery and the relief was wonderful. Barry and I talked long into the night about bringing her home, living through the challenges of the first few months or year of medical treatment and hospital visits, and being together with our older three children. My heart and arms ached to hold them and to be with them. Our family felt shattered into pieces, between hospital and home, between countries and cultures.

Several days later, I drowsed in the chair beside Beatrice's incubator. This is remarkable as the chair was desperately uncomfortable. It was made from hard slippery plastic, presumably so that it could be washed easily. However, when you relaxed into it, your body started to slip towards the floor. Resting in it required a delicate balance between relaxing and sitting upright. The room was still and warm, the nurse occasionally checking in on Beatrice and her roommate.

The third incubator was now empty.

A dark-haired woman in a fresh white coat came in, brought another chair over and sat down beside me. She looked sombre. 'Dr Quetille' was embroidered above the pocket of the coat. She introduced herself and offered to speak in English as she had something serious to talk about. My heart and mind immediately became submerged in an icy ocean of sorrow.

She was kind, and she gave the conversation plenty of time. She stopped several times to ask whether my husband could join me for the rest of the discussion. Each time I said no, he was not in France. I could see she was very uncomfortable with my being alone, but as I now guessed what was ahead, I urged her to continue speaking. Beatrice had had a devastating bleed in her brain. She would not survive this brain injury, or if she did, it would be 'a very dark future. Black. It will be a black future.'

She finished and sat back. I could no longer speak, just sat opposite her, destroyed. I'm sure she said many other things, but I heard nothing else. When I try to summon up the conversation, I remember little apart from her care, her kindness, her very definite message and the time she gave to it. I'll be for ever grateful for that. At the end of the exchange, she leant back in her chair, depleted. We sat together for a few moments in silence. She seemed reluctant to stand and leave. I never saw her again.

A year later, she and Dr Amolle wrote a letter to us, remembering Beatrice's birth and time in the NICU. The generosity of that letter stunned us and brought tears of sadness and love for two people in another country who had touched our lives too briefly. This letter, handwritten, captured perfectly how a seemingly small act can be the biggest act of all. In receiving that letter, we felt that Beatrice had been special to others, that she was remembered and that her name was said aloud by people who had known her.

On later reflection, I realised I had not asked Dr Quetille any questions about what exactly had happened. It seemed that the surgery had gone well, as the atmosphere that evening was light-hearted and positive. I did not ask why Beatrice had had a major bleed as the why would not change the what. I did not ask to see the results of blood tests or scans; I accepted the words as they were said and was not able to enquire any further. This was possibly because I was alone for the news. It's the only explanation I have for the absence of enquiry, or that I was too shocked at the prospect of Beatrice suffering for even a second longer. I'm not sure.

When Dr Quetille left the room, I thought of Barry, our children and the pain this news would bring them. I left the hospital and walked for hours in a daze, crying and stumbling, until eventually I had no energy left. It was only then that I was able to call my husband.

He took a flight the next day. Overnight Beatrice had begun to struggle to breathe on the ventilator, and now with more pain-relief medication, she seemed to be sleeping all the time. I held her perfect feet in my hands as I reached into the humid glass box she lived in. I closed my eyes. Under my fingers I could feel a tiny flutter, like the wings of a hummingbird. It was the fast thready pulse at her ankle.

Time stood still. How often I have summoned that memory back into my mind, a bittersweet balm on my longing.

A gentle chaplain offered to bless our baby. Hospital chaplains can be a much-needed emotional support to people, and I was glad this soft-spoken lady visited us in the NICU. Although neither of us had strong faith, the time we spent with her helped us. Clinging to our need to mark our daughter's presence in this world, we had a little baptism with her. We named our three children as godparents to Beatrice and stood in for them as the blessing was said. When I look back, I think it was at that point that acceptance and peace slipped into the room, and we knew we were not going to bring our tiny girl home to join her siblings.

Barry and I held Beatrice together until her heartbeat slowed and faded away. It was short, and yet it was long. It could never be long enough, and I wish she were here now, but it happened as it did. Nothing can change that.

I understand the simple solace of spending that time, to be part of the last breaths of a child who is cherished. I felt truly complete and blessed as a mother because I had the privilege of holding her warm body, and her soft face to mine, as her breath left and did not return. As her mother I had felt her growing inside me, I had heard one tiny cry when she was delivered, and I held her close on her last day. It was not enough, but I grasp at it like drops of water on my tongue after nineteen days in a desert. Beatrice had lived for nineteen sunny days and each one she was loved. That simple fact was a raft made of wreckage that I later clung to.

A young doctor slipped into the darkened room and rested her stethoscope on Beatrice's chest. She nodded and said softly in English, 'I am very sorry, your daughter is gone.' Then, just as quickly, she left the room.

We held Beatrice close until her body began to cool. This is very difficult to articulate. Your children have warm, vibrant bodies and they for ever feel part of your body. Holding Beatrice against my chest, I wanted the time never to end. We were quiet as there was no coherent thought that could be bashed into the shape of words. After some time, Barry put his hand on her little head and said, 'She isn't warm anymore,' and the realisation came into both of our heads that there was no way back. Until that point there was always the whisper of hope, that the message was wrong, that our child might recover. All our hopes and plans came to a searingly painful end in that NICU room, cradling our cold infant.

For some reason I never understood, we had to visit her the next morning in the hospital mortuary. It was set far apart from the main hospital building and took us ages to find. We trailed bleakly around in boiling hot sunshine, searching for it. Eventually, we found it: 'La Morgue'.

I deeply regret seeing my daughter in that dark, strange building. A slight man in a beige coat escorted us into a room almost entirely made of grey and green marble. His coat reminded me of the coats that bakers wore to deliver bread when I was a small child. The images before my eyes were dissociated in a chopped-up movie reel, making no sense.

Bewildered and afraid, we stood stock still in that bizarre mausoleum. The man returned with our daughter in a black box, similar to those used for filing cards in a library. Her name was written on a tiny piece of white card, inserted into the metal clip at the front. He lifted her out into Barry's arms. My gentle husband sobbed, hardly stopping to take a breath for himself. He keened. Our desolation was complete.

The image of her cold and stiff, dressed in baby clothes that were enormous on her tiny frame, burnt itself onto my retina and replaced all other images for a long time. It made me question everything I had felt for her, all the dreams I had had for her future. How could I have been so stupid to believe that she would live? I asked myself repeatedly, as that dreadful image swam in front of my eyes. I looked back on various comments her nurses had made over the three weeks and concluded that they had always known Beatrice was going to die, and that I was foolish for trotting in each day optimistically to see her. The throwing away of my breast milk came back to mind and signified everything I had missed in terms of understanding and felt like proof of my own naivety. My cruelty to her. My mind needled my broken person relentlessly in those early days, with the solitary thought that her death had been inevitable and that by agreeing to surgery I had selfishly prolonged her pain.

We flew back to Dublin the following afternoon. To arrive home without your baby, knowing you will never bring her home with you, is agony. To go out into the world having grown a child inside your body and not have that child with you creates visceral and mental anguish. Every moment I reminded myself of the hopeful plans I had made while sitting with her in the neonatal unit in a form of self-torture. We had dreamt of a life together and now it was gone. At home there were gifts of baby clothes and blankets, congratulations cards and feeding equipment. They sat in the house for close to a year before I could touch them.

My parents were taking care of our other children, so we drove to their house to collect them. My mother held me in a tight hug and rubbed my back in the warm way she had done for every other pain I had experienced. She never stopped recognising our loss in all the years that followed. Although my parents had never met or held their granddaughter, she was real to them, as they could see our love for her. I think this is the lens that needs to be held up to loss in other people – if you can see and feel the deep love and pain, you can bring to life the loss of the relationship and the person who is not there anymore.

Barry arranged for Beatrice to brought back for burial in Ireland. He was always a wonderful and capable father. On a surprisingly cold day at the end of the summer, I carried her slim white coffin into the church. When we later went to the graveyard and I placed her coffin carefully in the arms of the funeral director, he remarked on how light the coffin was. He said, 'Oh, my dear, how tiny she was.' He looked into my eyes and smiled slightly, saying, 'She is an innocent, a tiny butterfly.' The word 'innocent' stuck in my mind, and later when I looked up its meaning, I understood that Beatrice was not in our lives to bring pain. She was free from badness. She was goodness.

She rests now beside her grandfather, who never met her but would have welcomed her joyfully. They lie now in a plot surrounded by tall trees. Birds caw above and play in the ever-present wind that comes in from the sea, just over the hill. I don't feel their presence there. Instead I see and feel them in our generous and kind children.

Grief as a couple is complicated. Barry and I had to learn how to mourn our daughter separately, and bring those feelings together as a couple. On the day that Beatrice died I said to him, 'This will push us apart. We must fight against that.' He nodded and held me close. He did not waver from that promise. We walked together, sometimes on paths that diverged. Barry found solace in looking to the future and we viewed new houses to move into, new cars to replace our old one. We drifted to different ways of coping, with my mind turning backwards relentlessly. I spent hours creating a huge memory book of photos and reflections, remembrance cards to send to family and friends. There were weeks when it seemed we were both trying to get to the end of the journey but were following entirely different maps. Fortunately, we didn't lose sight of each other, although his path took him up barren mountains and mine went through a dark forest, where every tree looked the same and I was forever looking back over my shoulder.

Barry began to run long distances to help soothe his emotions. The world seemed filled with advertisements for nappies and follow-on milk, and everywhere we went, we saw new babies in buggies and glowing mothers with pregnant bellies. For many months these sights scalded us, like a touch on burnt skin.

The guilt I experienced during that time was crippling. The image of Beatrice lying cold and pale in the French mortuary came to my mind a thousand times each day, to be followed immediately by the thought, 'well, you didn't want her anyway.' I also blamed myself for the pain that my husband and children were experiencing. And then I would begin again the long list of I-should-haves, which grew longer every time I compiled it. The human mind can be a cage in which the darkest nights are lived, and it can feel impossible to escape. It has taken a thousand sleepless nights to forgive myself.

Our children brought such comfort during those months. The sensation of your arms being empty after the death of a baby is a powerful and primal force. Being able to hold my older children close to me soothed the ache. Barry and I immersed ourselves completely in the daily routines of school drop-off, swimming classes and reading bedtime stories. It was incredibly painful and awkward to interact with other people socially, and we withdrew from much of the wider circle around us. This wasn't intentional: it was just all too hard. Given the choice between going out and telling the terrible story again or staying at home and looking inwards, it was always less painful to make an excuse and stay at home.

Almost no one knew what to say. I remember hearing that statement about death long before our own experiences, and it returning to me after our daughter died. There were those I knew for decades who never mentioned my daughter's name or her passing. But it's more than just words that matter. Almost no one knew how to *be* with a bereaved mother. I found solace with several other mothers who had experienced the death of their baby.

Friends of friends reached out and distinguished themselves with their own loss. They understood the value of acknowledging the loss. They knew to use Beatrice's name, and to ask questions about Beatrice's life and the dreams we had had for her. They knew that in saying her name, she lived on. Their own difficult days had gifted them with the courage to speak about being a mother to their baby who died, or who had been taken away from them. One beautiful woman in her eighties wrote to me about the death of two of her babies and how she had never lost the need to acknowledge those children, although they lay in unmarked graves. Perhaps arising out of our conversations over the next couple of years, she decided to add their names to the headstone she had engraved on her husband's grave.

Loss softens, but it does not disappear.

Each week I took one of my children to a music class and sat waiting outside with a woman and her new baby. We had been pregnant at the same time just months earlier and had exchanged smiles and some chat as our bumps grew over the weeks, as winter became spring.

In the autumn term of music, she fed her baby sitting so close I could smell her perfume. I could smell her milk. As her baby grumbled and latched on for a feed, my breasts ached, and my body flooded with loss. There was a physical vulnerability that existed in addition to the emotional. I would steel myself before each class and button up my emotions so that I would not betray the depth of my despair. Inside my mind, I was lying at her feet howling. Outside, I smiled benignly and asked how she was doing. The feelings were not of resentment or a desire to take her baby from her arms. I wanted to feel my breasts tingle with the cry of my own child, to lift her from her buggy and snuggle her onto my body with the fierce and natural connection that being mother to a new baby gives. To feel the peace and contentment that feeding a baby into a satiated slumber offers to the lucky parent who has been chosen to care. My body desired this connection, though my mind knew it was not possible.

As the term finished at Christmas in the music class, and parents waiting to pick up their children wished each other a happy break, the new mother turned to me and said, 'I hope you have a lovely time with your family, especially as it's your baby's first Christmas.' She had obviously assumed that I didn't usually bring the baby to collect my older children.

I blurted out, 'My baby died.'

The woman looked horrified and glanced down protectively to her little one in her arms. 'Oh, I'm so sorry, I didn't know,' she replied.

'It's OK,' I said sadly. When I saw her in the new year, she looked embarrassed and dipped her gaze away from me. I couldn't make it all right, and we never spoke again.

Almost a year after Beatrice had died, I went to a dinner party and dear friends with good intentions put a new baby into my arms at the table. I sat frozen, looking at his perfect face, and thought that my heart could not be more broken than it was right then. I was too embarrassed to say how I felt as I believed no one would understand that I was still grieving. In the throes of grief, I had hung my own giant clock on the wall. Beatrice was in our lives so briefly, and it was now a year later. I was way behind where I should have been. When I was able to recall that evening, after a lot of time had passed and I felt stronger, I could see that my friends would never have judged my sorrow in that way. But I did not speak. So they did not know.

Though I was drowning in the dark sea of sorrow, I appeared to be swimming along nicely in a perfect front crawl. But I no longer knew who I was. I had no identity, and no connection to who I had been before Beatrice, and no ability to connect with the future. These were the blackest moments, when I thought that if I stopped existing it would not make any difference to anyone, as there was no 'I'.

In fact, I reasoned, 'I' was already gone.

This erosion of identity I did not understand. I was a clear windowpane that I observed almost at a distance. It frightened me enormously. But it also consoled me, as I decided that it would be a relief to all when they finally saw that I was gone. Unlike Sylvia Plath, who seemed resigned as she described herself as being a ghostly flower flat as paper and flat of colour, I felt a raw terror as I was pulled closer to oblivion.

It is not possible to come to terms with the loss of unconditional love. It is not possible to recover. Fighting against that reality led to my own disappearance. I stopped washing or caring for my body. I slept in my clothes and wore the same things day after day. When Barry gently asked why, I replied that I was cold. I was too cold to care about anything that wasn't my remaining three children.

My children, who are now older, like to poke fun at me for my facial expression in a family photo taken when we were on a roller-coaster some years ago. While they sit around me, smiling with their arms out to embrace the wild fun of the ride, I sit with my head down. Resembling a medieval gargoyle, my face is screwed up in agony. My eyes are obliterated, they are squeezed so tightly shut against the experience. That is the same position I took when thrown into the shock of grief. I took a deep breath in and closed my eyes and my heart. If that deep breath brought me to cold calm and the end of my painful existence, so be it.

I had a fear that if I started speaking about how much pain I felt and my fight to quell it, I would never be able to put it all back together afterwards. I was a mother, a wife and a doctor. At all times I expected myself to hold everything together. Other people in my life expected me to hold things together. Nothing else was acceptable to me.

Barry and I decided to go to counselling. I don't recall that decision, so I think he must have guided me to it. At the beginning I experienced bottomless horror at speaking about how I felt, panic at opening the gate to the feelings that would inevitably follow the words. Although I had been present at the death of many patients, I knew nothing about the power of grief, and I had no understanding that its force could demolish me as a person.

The first counselling session did not go well. We went to a group meeting in a community centre, which, in retrospect, I see that I was in no way ready for. When it came to our turn to speak, I could say no words. Barry spoke for us.

Everyone else spoke. They told the stories of their loss and how they felt now. I felt a pang of ease as it appeared that I would be able to leave the session without opening my mouth. I may even have relaxed my guard slightly, which was my undoing.

As the facilitator went around the circle a second time, a woman sitting opposite me spoke about her teenager who had taken their own life. The depth of despair in her voice pulled at a thread of the weighted blanket I had hidden my feelings under. I began to cry. In the shallow water of my mind, I was crying because the stranger in a pink fluffy sweater directly across the room from me was so incredibly sad. The kind facilitator couldn't help me and, although the other parents in the group were sympathetic and leant towards me in comfort, I could not stop crying. Barry almost carried me out of the room.

Now there was a new narrative in my head – the world was a terrible place, there was only sorrow, and I was beyond help. It would be only a matter of time before everyone else realised this and let me slip away.

Almost mute during the day, at night I woke screaming because I couldn't find the baby in our bed. I had a recurring dream that I had been feeding Beatrice in my arms and had fallen asleep and somehow dropped her under the blankets. On waking in the dream, I pulled and grabbed at the duvet, searching desperately for my baby. Screaming at Barry to help find her. He held me until I woke properly and then we cried together, broken again at the realisation that another day had begun. The push and pull of emotional tides, dragging our bodies towards each other and apart again. Scrabbling at the bottom of this ocean, trying to find Beatrice.

It was a dark time.

With my husband's support I returned to individual bereavement counselling. With time, some light returned: we began to talk to each other and share understanding and warmth again. We moved into a common experience and conversation where we simply stopped trying to recover. We instead spoke about the fact that Beatrice was not with us, but she could remain alive in our words and feelings. This subtle change freed us both. It is not possible to capture how testing it is to grieve singly and together, except to say that we were never the same couple again. This is because we were not the same people we were before our daughter died. There were new strengths to this altered space that we shared, and there were new insights into each other, some difficult and some good.

Any energy we had we devoted to the three young children we had always adored and now cherished with a ferocity that blocked out anyone else. We had a heightened sense of protection for them, and certainly for years after Beatrice died, I struggled with waves of panic that something terrible would happen to them. To this day, that dread swims deep.

As we healed as a family, the fog began to lift, and my thoughts became clearer. I did not travel in and out of anger or bargaining when immersed in grief for Beatrice. I have since learnt that each loss in your life is experienced entirely differently. Some of the landscape is familiar, but the whirl of emotion has a different hue each time. With my defenceless daughter, whom I felt I had not always loved and protected, my grief was characterised by sorrow, regret and a profound disconnection from myself. Shame at being a mother found wanting drove much of that separation.

The events that had occurred seemed so empty of purpose. Why us? Why was Beatrice conceived if she was only to be born too early and die? The only meaning that I could give her painfully brief existence was that I should create significance and meaning with her life and death.

I was in the gym one morning, shortly before the end of my maternity leave, sitting on the rowing machine, pulling back and forth. My thoughts kept me disconnected from the lulling movement of the machine, but the physical exertion was comforting.

I gazed straight ahead, past the top of the rowing machine, and with crystal clarity, I saw it.

There was a choice in front of me. It had been there on the road for years and years, like a dusty exit sign for a forgotten destination, but for some reason I had not seen it. Beatrice's life and death and all we experienced individually, as a couple and as a family, shone a light on that road sign and the message emblazoned upon it. I should return to work in paediatric intensive care and bring our experiences with me.

We had lived through a challenging pregnancy, medical care through a language and culture not our own, surgery on our precious daughter, complications, her untimely death, profound grief and questioning. If I returned to the fires that had smelted and cast us as statues of loss, we might live it again, but differently. Our loss would power love and understanding for other parents. We could be new in purpose. Every day I could carry our tiny daughter, tucked up in my heart, and work in a way that honoured her goodness and her brief life.

It had been almost a decade since I had worked full-time in PICU. Since completing my fellowship training at PICU in Australia I had been working predominantly as a consultant in anaesthesiology. Although closely related specialties, they are different in some important ways. I contacted my former colleagues in the PICU from years ago and asked if I could be considered for a post in paediatric intensive-care medicine. They knew how much I had loved the work in the past. With their support, I left my post as an anaesthesiologist in mixed adult and paediatric practice, where I had previously been content, and returned to PICU.

Would I have broken with the tradition of staying in a senior permanent post and gone back to the beginning had Beatrice never existed? I don't believe I would.

Without question it was the right thing to do. There remains a bridge between my experience with Beatrice and my love of caring for sick children and children at the end of their lives. They are inextricable and one could not exist without the other.

With meaning, so much loss and pain are bearable.

Even more than bearable.

In meaning, there is hope.

17. Words

'Words are events, they do things, change things. They transform both the speaker and hearer; they feed energy back and forth and amplify it. They feed understanding or emotion back and forth and amplify it.'

Ursula K. Le Guin

A new chapter began in our lives in 2014 as I returned to work full-time in intensive care. Almost ten years had passed since I had left it, and I now felt a different person. A mother, a wife, a doctor and a bereaved parent.

Back in PICU, one of the first things I noticed was the different way in which words mattered. Maya Angelou once spoke about how it's not the words spoken but how a person makes us feel that creates a lasting impression. This is never truer than the first conversations with parents when their child is admitted to hospital. Years later the words said will drift in memory, but a feeling of warmth and understanding will persist.

Yet the words matter. They are vitally important and will be recalled in snippets and phrases. It's not a contradiction:

words must be tailored perfectly to the child and their family, but emphasis must also lie in the non-verbal communication as it creates the lasting memory of being respected and cared for.

The words said have a purpose beyond the communication of a diagnosis or a clinical status. They take life by helping a family create a narrative. Later this will become part of the child's story – the story of them when they were sick. Mostly in the PICU we have a reasonable sense of where the child's progress will take them and their family, but occasionally it's more uncertain.

Being honest in the narrative is key. Ideally it is one of hope, tempered with realistic expectations, to hold everyone through what could be a long journey. In contrast to caring for an adult who is critically ill, and possibly at the end of their life, it's usually not possible to find out what the child's wishes or goals of care are or their priorities when time is short. The goals of care are what the parents express, and generally the goal is the continuation of life. It is woven into the genetic code of parents to desire quantity of life, as well as quality, for their child. There is no word for a bereaved parent. They are not a widow or widower; there is no word because it shouldn't exist. Acceptance of inevitable death in a baby or child is immeasurably difficult for their parents.

As physicians and as nurses, we must be guides. We are the sherpa who must put the heavy burden on our back and face up to the black craggy mountain, as we draw a cloak around the shivering, frightened people who have been forced to climb up through the blizzard. As we climb together, we tell a story. It is our duty to place a stake in the ice with a message that we may need to return to. If we need to go back to this marker, we must together find a message of hope.

Becky had been sick for a few days before her mum, Fionnuala, brought her to the emergency department. She had asthma and every winter would get a nasty lung infection that took weeks to shake off. Fionnuala thought this was the same. Becky had a chromosomal abnormality called trisomy 21, commonly referred to as Down Syndrome. She was eight years old and the life and soul of her class in primary school, which made it even more disturbing to see her on an emergency department trolley, listless and grunting for air. As she took each fast, shallow breath, her head bobbed forward with the effort it took to shift air in and out of her lungs. Her oxygen levels were falling, which was making her agitated, so she wouldn't allow the oxygen mask to stay on her face.

Every time the nurse looked up at the vital signs on the wall monitor and frowned, she moved the mask onto Becky's face – and immediately Becky swiped it off. The nurse pointed at the red rash that was spreading across Becky's chest. It looked angry, the patches merging with each other. The nurse turned to me and raised her eyebrows. I shook my head. I didn't know what the rash meant. She drew me to the side and said, 'I think this is measles.'

Fionnuala looked stressed, sitting beside her daughter. 'This isn't like her,' she repeated several times. 'She's normally as good as gold when we visit the doctor. . .' When a sick child has a chronic medical issue in the background, the parents frequently strive to make their usual level of

105

function or behaviour clear to the staff who are assessing their child. They fear that what they see as different and worrying in their child will not be noticed by the staff caring for them.

We explained to Fionnuala that Becky showed several worrying signs that made admission to the PICU the safest course over the next few hours. There, a little later, it became clear that Becky was deteriorating further and was not going to manage on a tight-fitting mask and ventilator to help her breathing.

I sat outside Becky's room with Fionnuala and Becky's father, Niall. I showed them the X-ray of her lungs, which now resembled a snowstorm across both lung fields. We were suspicious that Becky had an infection with the measles virus. 'What can you do for this?' asked Niall.

'There is no specific treatment unfortunately,' I said. 'We must support Becky's body to heal itself.' They nodded, Fionnuala turning away to peer through the window of the room to where her daughter lay in bed. I could see silent tears sliding down the side of her face.

I asked her about Becky's vaccines as a baby. 'I think we missed the MMR,' she said. 'Becky was a real worry when she was small, and I was afraid of the MMR . . .' Her voice disappeared to a whisper. She covered her face with her hands and sobbed.

'Becky is a healthy little girl, and she has fought her way through other health problems,' I continued, dropping seeds into the story. 'We would expect her to fight her way through this, although there may be setbacks and some very difficult days.'

106

Fionnuala turned back to face me. 'Yes,' she said. 'Becky is a fighter.' The narrative of Becky being critically sick had begun.

That evening we sedated Becky, and she was placed, anaesthetised, on a ventilator. The ventilator settings increased gradually as the hours went by, her nurse suctioning a tide of thick green secretions from her lungs. Her temperature shot up and we struggled to bring it down to the normal range. In the small hours of the morning, we had to change ventilators to one that moved the lungs in a different fashion, holding them open continuously. Her blood pressure fell as the pressure on her heart increased. In just eight hours, she had gone from being lethargic in her mother's car, to utterly dependent on life-sustaining medical equipment.

The following day involved chasing samples that had been sent to the laboratory for analysis, to focus our treatment better. We did as much imaging of Becky's organs at the bedside as we could: moving her to the radiology department would have been perilous. Becky's little face, still full of freckles from the summer holidays months earlier, had become swollen and pale. We gave her a transfusion of red blood cells to try to carry more oxygen to her tissues that were besieged with infection.

I gave Niall and Fionnuala an update on where we were, beginning, 'Where do you think we are right now with Becky's illness?'

Niall shook his head. They both looked exhausted. 'Is she going to die?' he asked, looking directly into my eyes.

'We now know that Becky has a severe measles infection and that there is also a significant bacterial infection in her lungs, which we should know more about tomorrow,' I replied. I knew I wasn't answering his question. The facts were important to them, but the message they needed was not based in numbers or clinical data. 'Becky's body is fighting this. We can see signs that her immune system is rising to the challenge. That's good. Even though she is extremely ill now, there are some positive signs. It's too early to say much more, but we are all optimistic that she will get through this,' I finished, standing up.

Fionnuala reached over, took my hand and squeezed it, saying, 'Thank you for being honest. We're very grateful to all of you.'

The next two days were tense, as Becky's kidneys became weaker and could not clear the fluid that now gathered in all her tissues. We conferred as a team and agreed that to keep her lungs functioning enough to carry out acceptable gas exchange, we would have to commence dialysis to assist her kidneys in removing fluid from her body. Needing dialysis was not completely surprising but at the same time we were disappointed and anxious about the need to escalate her organ support even further. We were now supporting four of her organ systems with technology and medications, which substantially altered her chances of survival.

The nursing shift leader, Cathal, and I sat with Becky's parents, and we went through the facts and our reasons for adding dialysis to the intensive-care supports. I checked to see if they had any questions for us. They shook their heads without saying anything. These conversations are enormous in significance and overwhelming in emotion. It's almost impossible to distil even a single question that could answer the swirling maelstrom of terror.

I closed my eyes as we sat in silence absorbing where we were just then, and I felt their pain. It clutched my heart, tight and uncomfortable. That kind of pain makes you wonder if you will take another breath and comes with a feeling of panic.

I opened my eyes and invited them to say how they were feeling about the information we had imparted. It wasn't enough to help them speak. All types of reactions to bad news are understood, tears, anger, silence, but handing over the opportunity to question, to articulate terror is important. Although I recall Becky clearly, the reality is that I will not think about her every day of my remaining years. Depending on the events in those fragile hours and how we held them, Niall and Fionnuala might think about it every day for ever. There was no space for judgement, only empathy.

Becky's nurse Aoife had been caring for her for the last two days and had come to know the family a little more. As Fionnuala and Niall sat in silence, grappling with the information we had given them, Aoife spoke. 'Becky sounds like a strong little girl. She hasn't let her other medical issues stop her playing rugby – amazing!'

Niall smiled a little. 'That's true,' he said. 'She's a demon on the pitch.'

We laughed at the idea of Becky in the thick of the action. In that split second of shared humour there was the connection we needed to bring everyone back to the present, back to Becky. 'And you two have got her to where she is in school and in her sports,' I added, looking at them with encouragement. 'Although we are all very worried about Becky, we've got to keep going here.' I paused, then made my voice even more serious. 'We will tell you if we think we have no further treatments for Becky and that she is not going to recover. We will try to give you time. But we are not at that point now.' Again, they looked anxious, but they nodded with apparent understanding. 'We'll stay optimistic for now,' I concluded.

Becky recovered. Her lungs cleared of fluid and infection gradually and we were able to stop dialysis. Her blood pressure and heart rate settled towards normal for her age, and her gut began to absorb and digest food.

She woke up with a bang just as the day shift commenced, about three weeks after her admission. Her nurse called her parents, and they arrived in time to see their daughter sitting up. Her eyes were open, and she gestured at the breathing tube, asking for it to be removed. A little later that morning the tube was taken out. Becky was hoarse and her voice was weak, but her face was a delight as she snuggled into Fionnuala's arms.

That afternoon, as Becky's physiotherapist Annmarie was working with her, I joined her parents to use words to paint the picture of what the next weeks were likely to bring. I pulled over a chair and sat beside them as Annmarie gently encouraged Becky to move her limbs, sit to the side of the bed and stand for a few seconds. Again, I mentioned potential setbacks and issues that might prove surprisingly challenging.

I got the feeling that they were both so mesmerised with the leap in progress Becky had made they were not listening to my cautious explanation of the next steps. Still, most of the messaging over the preceding weeks had been sufficient to guide them across the mountain pass. More of Becky's story would be created the next day, and the day after that. Had her illness taken a different direction and she had deteriorated to a point beyond recovery, we would have kindly used every support and communication tool possible to try to bring peaceful acceptance to her parents. Becky would have lived her life to the full, surrounded by love, and she would have died in gentle comfort with her family around her.

The words would have been different. Her story would have been a different kind of inspiration.

All stories contain that potential for inspiration.

18. Clean Pyjamas

'The secret in caring for the patient is in caring for the patient.'

Francis Peabody

Most mornings before work, my husband and I had break-fast together. It was always very early, before the children woke up. It made for a gentle start, with him emptying the dishwasher and me finishing the lunchboxes for school. We wouldn't necessarily chat much, but it was a precious time when we were aligned in our view of the day ahead. Then we sat at our kitchen table and sipped tea while listening to the morning news on the radio.

If there was a report about a child being injured overnight in a car accident, or some other event, we would fall silent. Any mention of a house fire on the morning news gives me an icy dread in the pit of my stomach. My ears will prick up to find out where it was and whether there were any people in the house. Any children.

There's no other way to put this: injury or death in a house fire is horrible. When called into the emergency department and a small boy is lying on the trolley, caked in sticky black dirt, the fear and smell of burning filth and flesh assaults every one of your senses.

Like Paul.

Paul had been the last child retrieved from a house fire by the fire crew. Several adults and a baby had managed to escape or be helped out earlier. It was 5 a.m. It seems necessary for it to be 5 a.m. for this kind of horror. I had been called in from home and stood at the head of the bed and watched a large fireman carry Paul in. The man had streaks down his dusty face. They may have been tears. A garda officer comforted a young paramedic who looked utterly broken. The room was quiet otherwise.

Paul was alive. But his oxygen levels were seriously low and there were many other worrying features. We sorted our main tasks to stabilise him as best we could and took him up to the PICU. For the following few hours, it wasn't possible to improve his oxygen stores, and his brain showed signs that it was dying. All that sticky melted plastic was coating the inside of his lungs and the poison had seeped into every cell.

His dad, also Paul, hadn't been in the house fire. Families are complicated and change shape over the years. Children inhabit the folds of these arrangements.

Big Paul came in to sit with little Paul. We explained that his tiny little namesake was going to die today. We have sat with hundreds, maybe even thousands, of people and said the words that destroy their world. It does not get easier.

'He's my best little bud.' He shook his head. 'He goes in the van with me, real early like, and we do the deliveries.

113

Who's going to sit in the van with me now?' He choked on the last words, that question. He used language in such a down-to-earth way to describe a little boy, held each day in the unconditional love of his father, that I could see my own boys and their father in the image. That question of what we do when our world is torn down.

For the next few hours, big Paul sat and talked to little Paul. He spoke to him without stopping, about their days together, what they liked to do, where they went. We carried on with our work, listening to big Paul's voice telling little Paul that they'd be back out on the road in no time.

Little Paul's heart slowed and stopped beating. I lifted him into his father's arms, and we all hugged each other. Everyone cried. Big Paul had painted a picture in such detail of their normal moments as boy and dad bound together that each one of us could see the massive hole left behind in this man's life as little Paul left.

The nurses washed little Paul. They talked to him too. They talked about the blue sky outside, the trees coming into cherry blossom, summer holidays and cartoons on the telly. Nurses know how to wash a child's body lovingly, continuing dignity and humanity into death. Once I asked Julie, one of our nurses, how they knew to do this. How did they know to talk to the person as if they were still there?

'It's just what we do,' I was told simply, with a shrug of her shoulders and slight bemused dismissal that it was anything to be asking about.

As a child I lived in a town where it was uncommon for people to be laid out after death at home, so I didn't grow up among women who knew what to do. From the time I was an intern, being called to wards to verify death, I have been drawn to the rituals that nurses carry out to honour the remains of a human. The cleansing, the soothing and the dressing. It is a shadowy world that doctors are not part of.

We had no pyjamas for a child of Paul's size, so our healthcare assistant Ger dipped into the kitty and went to the nearest shop to buy some. We wanted big Paul to see and hold his little son with his hair washed clear of soot, his beautiful face shining and clean Paw Patrol jammies. This is the pride and love that goes with caring for small children no matter where the day has taken the child and their family. When I had sat listening to the radio that morning, immersed in the comfort of my home, I had no clue that this was where the day would go.

The love and special care that is lavished on each child is for them and for their family. But it's also for us. We must take our work to the best possible conclusion, in the most awful circumstances, and feel that we have done so. There is a glimmer of peace in the pride wrought out of pain.

It's the only way it is possible to say goodbye and then go to the next child.

19. Believe It Can Happen

'If you feel pain, you are alive. And if you feel other people's pain, you are a human being.'

Leo Tolstoy

One of the intimate privileges of caring for tiny sick babies was the restoration of personal hope after our own daughter died. After coming back to work in the PICU, the first baby I met who was admitted for the same surgery Beatrice had had floored me completely. Here was an infant who had a chance, with his parents who were full of hope.

I was intent on delivering medical care that would optimise his opportunity to recover after surgery. When I took the baby's tiny head into my hands to reposition his breathing tube, I focused on the details of the task and the next steps needed to prepare him for the operating room. I swallowed the swirl of emotions that threatened to overwhelm me until I had time a few days later to walk on the beach.

Solitude wasn't possible with a husband and children, so on a bitterly cold Sunday afternoon I took my daughters to the beach where I had grown up. I set them the job of throwing the ball for our dog and I sat on the sea wall watching them. They were wrapped in layers of sweaters and hats, their little faces pink in the cold air. It was then that I could finally set out my thoughts and feelings on the care of premature babies. In an analytical frame of mind initially, I tried deliberately to shift my thoughts from regrets and what-ifs to the reasons I had returned to work in a PICU: because I could make a tiny difference, and because I could use our experiences to help others.

It was difficult to ignore the wish that each baby who recovered was mine. That could never be. A wave of emotion broke with the image of my hand holding the baby's earlier in the week, just as I had held my daughter's. My grief and self-recrimination rushed back, freezing my mind. I panicked at the prospect of tumbling back into the paralysis that had clutched me before. I stared hard at the stony ground in front of me. Then, like the different coloured pebbles under my feet, I saw the thousands of hands I had touched over the years since becoming a doctor. In that visualisation I found self-compassion. The babies I would care for offered renewed hope to everyone around them, not only their family. Each one was a seed of good things that might happen. Just as Beatrice was and continues to be. It was kinder and wiser to choose to be part of that hopeful purpose than to turn away from it.

We left the grey skies of January and the beach and returned home. My heart felt sore, a muscle that had contracted hard to pull through. But I knew it as a constructive pain that would gain me strength.

Babies born early confront us with potential sadness and hope. I chose to see optimism and would make that choice again every day. When a baby is born early, they could be weeks being cared for in a neonatal intensive-care unit, making good progress. The shock of admission fades a little for their parents, and they start to make new routines around their growing infant. If a complication such as a bowel perforation or a heart issue develops, there is a new round of shock and loss of grip on where and what the parents believe everything to be. A second round of upheaval is a very challenging time for new mothers and fathers.

Baby Angie was referred to us by a neonatologist in another hospital. She had been making steady progress since she was born at only twenty-four weeks – four months early. She had been gaining weight, fed with her mother's breast milk through a tube from her nose to her stomach, as her suck hadn't developed. She was lively and already had a special, feisty character.

Now twenty-eight weeks, Angie had become breathless, and her heart was struggling with more work to do: a blood vessel between her heart and her lungs had stayed open. It is a connecting vessel, vital when a baby is growing inside their mother and the placenta is doing all the work of the lungs. It should naturally close in the days after birth, when the baby's lungs are open and carrying out the important business of bringing oxygen into the bloodstream and clearing carbon dioxide. The team in the NICU had been treating the vessel with medication, which frequently helps it to close. In Angie, it did not close and put pressure on her heart.

The cardiologist who had been reviewing her became increasingly concerned about this and asked us to accept transfer from the NICU. It was a busy week, and we didn't have a bed available. The shift leader Colette added Angie's name to the list of patients requiring PICU admission. Each morning the NICU called us, and each morning we had to ask them to wait. Without a doubt, this added to the emotional demand on everyone, especially Angie's parents, Jim and Allie. Now that they knew their tiny daughter needed an intervention to close the troublesome blood vessel, they naturally wanted it carried out as soon as possible. They believed it stood in the way of her getting back on track with her feeding and developing. It was a tense time.

Finally, we had enough capacity to take Angie from the NICU. She arrived by ambulance, bundled up in an incubator and accompanied by a medical transport team of five trained paramedics, doctors and nurses. They surrounded Angie, carefully lifting their precious cargo out of the incubator. She weighed a bit shy of a kilogram.

We started to get her ready for her procedure, which was planned for the next morning. Jim and Allie were waiting outside anxiously to see Angie in her new environment. When they came in, they were upset. Nothing was right, everything was different, and the tension was unbearable as they were clearly struggling not to explode at the nurse who was caring for Angie.

The shift leader asked my consultant colleague Sandra to sit with them for a few minutes. She invited them to share their worries, sat quietly and listened. The room was too noisy, they said; Angie liked her incubator set warmer; too many people were touching her; they didn't know where to bring Allie's breast milk; they were waiting too long outside before they could come in ... words tumbled out in a heated tangle. They spoke more and more, as they could see that they were being listened to and believed. Allie started to cry.

'We understand how frightening this is for you. We'll take care of Angie,' said Sandra. 'And as soon as she's ready, we'll send her back to the NICU,' she went on. 'Would you like that?' she asked, with a smile. Allie nodded, her sobs starting to ease.

Allie and Jim had been trying to have a baby together for seven years. They had walked the lonely road of IVF four times, blood tests, injections, counting eggs and embryos, and trying to cling to the belief that they would be parents. Angie was their first baby born alive. It was incomprehensible and terrifying to them that she had hit this speed bump in her progress. Now, as the risks of surgery and anaesthesia were explained to them, they were frightened she might be snatched away from them for ever.

The state of shock at the time of her early birth had returned, and it was a long night before Angie's transfer to the operating room. The exhausted couple walked to the operating room with the incubator and Nas, their nurse. Minutes later they returned to PICU to start the awful wait while the procedure was performed. Nas took them to our parents' sitting room and sat with Allie and Jim while they showed her photos of Angie and little videos they had made of her over the preceding weeks. Then they showed her messages they had had from friends and family and told her about Allie's pregnancy. It was the time and empathy they needed to soak themselves in the rich tapestry of images already present in their lives because of Angie. The kindness of the nurse that morning brought out the good things that had happened since Allie had become pregnant with Angie, and her birth.

I knew that Nas was meant to go on her rest break while Angie was in the operating room – but she never said a word about that to Jim and Allie. Instead, she sat with them and gave everything she could. Empathy is the cupped hand around a waning flame of belief, protecting it from the icy wind and helping it burn stronger.

Angie's surgery was a lovely success. The blood vessel was closed with a tiny device shaped like Mary Poppins's umbrella. She returned to the PICU, and we followed her closely, monitoring her for changes in her heart function and breathing. A couple of hours later she had become so much stronger that we made the decision to transfer her back that evening to the NICU.

'She's done so well, we're going to send your little lady back to her first circle of admirers,' I told her parents. They joined in the smiles around Angie's incubator, with deep breaths of relief.

The medical transport team returned. In the twenty-four hours since they had left us, they had been to three different hospitals, bringing babies to where they could get the treatment they required. Without question, their energy for the task was unique. They swept Angie into the transport pod and said their goodbyes. Jim and Allie hugged us all and thanked us. Jim dipped his head a bit and looked sheepish. 'We just stopped believing in you all for a minute. I'm sorry,' he said, referring to their restrained anger and unhappiness the day before.

'We understand. We really do,' I replied, looking him in the eye.

'Send us a photo of Angie when you go home,' called Nas, as they left.

Allie waved brightly. 'Oh, you'd better believe it.' She laughed. 'We'll send you photos of Angie every week till you beg us to stop!'

Every parent should feel that relief, that restoration back on the narrow path facing into the sun. Tempered with the knowledge and experience that it could be stolen at any moment, the swell of joy lifts the chin.

20. The Gift of Time

'All we have to decide is what to do with the time that is given us.'

J.R.R. Tolkien

Some people need more time. More time than the average patient, more time than the last patient, more time than the journals and textbooks tell us to expect. On an intellectual level we know this, but it can be a struggle to weather the time when uncertainty and worry about undue suffering and harm nip at us each day.

We had weekly meetings about Sandeep to provide an overview of where his prognosis and current treatment were and an update on how his family were coping with his long admission in the PICU. The value of our collective experience in different international centres, over a cumulative period of decades, is really felt during these meetings.

But we were flummoxed by Sandeep. He had a cancer diagnosis, and dozens of complications had occurred at every stage of his treatment. Each of those complications, such as infection or bleeding from his bladder or clots in his leg blood vessels, had taken weeks to treat and get him back on course with the overall goal of clearing the cancer cells from his body. We were incredibly conscious that, in the meantime, a small boy was losing ground from a developmental, social and psychological perspective. 'Where were we going with this?' we asked ourselves and each other.

So, another cycle of investigations began, following discussion with Sandeep's parents and the numerous teams now involved in his care. Ultrasound scans, bone-marrow aspirates, specialised genetic and infection screening tests that must be sent abroad for analysis. Those investigations had the silent function of gifting more time, as the test results must be awaited, then interpreted.

One of our PICU registrars, Liz, had formed a special relationship with Sandeep and his family. She spoke passionately at each handover round that she was certain Sandeep was interacting more with everyone and getting stronger. There was little objective evidence of the recovery Liz described. I reflected on patients who had touched me in a special way when I was in training and thought she was experiencing a similar wish to will a child better. I remembered feeling it too. When she spoke, I felt it again. The spirit of human connection and belief in a good outcome is a vital part of working in critical-care medicine. It should be cherished, not crushed with cynicism or bitterness.

Liz was correct. Sandeep had begun to stir under the blankets of support and treatments, a weak and sleepy bear emerging from hibernation. His complications dissipated. He was able to manage with less and less technology to help him breathe and began more intensive rehabilitative treatment. Annmarie, our physiotherapist, devised a programme of exercises and activities to tackle every muscle. Sandeep's mother, Mirha, added other elements to the plan, so there was time each day for cuddles on her lap, reading, ice-cream eating and washing, which they did together as a family. It was endearing to see Mirha guide Sandeep's weak, skinny arms up to wash her face with a flannel as he giggled at the funny expressions she made.

There were happy grins and waves from all the staff out on the floor as Sandeep left his room twice a day, initially in a recumbent wheelchair and later with a supported tricycle. He did laps around the PICU, with his equipment in tow, his nurse and physiotherapist encouraging him. His legs were wasted away to little sticks, and he could barely reach the pedals with his feet, but he knew when he was getting ready to go out for a 'walk' and his smile and huge bright eyes told everyone that nothing would stop him. The PICU registrar who had advocated optimism on Sandeep's darkest days had a permanent 'I told you so' cheeriness about her, which was heartening to witness.

Eventually, after four months of treatment for problems that had been numerous and often poorly understood, Sandeep was strong and stable enough to be discharged to the oncology ward. There he continued his treatment for cancer.

Six months later, Mirha and Sandeep walked into the PICU. They were going home that day and had come up to say thank you to the whole critical-care team. He still looked frail but had regained some weight and his hair was starting to grow in tufts above his ears. He was in remission and life could begin again. The clock had been reset to happier times.

Our family had benefited from the passage of time too.

Time had blurred the sharp edges of the grief we had experienced after Beatrice had left us. Arthur, Estella and Dorothea were thriving, and daily life was full to the brim. Then time presented us with a gift.

I got pregnant against the odds, as I was now forty-three.

Every antenatal visit, I exchanged nervous looks with our obstetrician as he scanned the growing baby. He was tense, and I knew then that Beatrice's death had distressed him, too. Although having another child after everything that had happened did not make sense to some people, our doctor and midwives never questioned it. That meant a lot to us, as the feelings during a pregnancy that come after a loss, or after multiple losses, are complicated.

Charles was born healthy and almost at term on a soft September morning. His hair glowed gold with red tips. He quickly made his place as the youngest in the nest, and from the moment he arrived, it felt like he had always been there. Babies who arrive after the death of a child are sometimes called 'rainbow' babies. They never replace the one who died: that is simply not possible. But their presence draws light back into a family, a stripe of colour and warmth after a brutal storm.

21. Witness

'One word frees us of all the weight and pain in life. That word is love.'

Sophocles

Not every day in intensive care is filled with drama. Some pass almost without notice, and it can be important to remind everyone that these are valuable, too. A quiet day in the unit allows patients stability, and staff some space to reflect. These are the days that stack up into years.

There was nothing more wonderful than to slip out of work a little early and join other parents in the gallery at the swimming pool where my children were taking classes or to appear unannounced at the side of a hockey pitch. I could never promise to be there, due to the unknown nature of each day. Barry's working hours were more predictable, so he was the more reliable parent in terms of showing up at the school.

One particularly gentle day, when I thought I might make it to swimming, changed in a second. That's the way this work goes.

The cardiac arrest happened abruptly yet was not entirely unexpected. This is a contradiction. Abigail was a cardiac patient and was critically sick, but stable. Another contradiction. The lack of sense lies in the fact that Abigail's heart was beating weakly, and we were racing against the clock to intervene – but it was always likely that we would lose the race. Our tools were puny compared to the disease that wreaked destruction on the muscle of Abigail's heart. The sand in the hourglass ran through before we had traced any other options. There were no other options. Abigail's heart stopped.

We leapt into action to get it beating again. Resuscitation efforts are always noisy and disruptive to the normal working day. There's no soft and mellow way to persuade a heart to start pumping again. Instead teams of people were arriving, more machines being wheeled in, phones and bleeps ringing, medication orders being shouted and alarms sounding. As we poured our own hearts into bringing that girl back into life, I glanced up across the room and, through the window, I saw Johnny.

Johnny was twelve years old. He was sitting in a chair beside his own PICU bed, drips and drains dotted around his pale body. His big eyes were transfixed on Abigail and all that was happening around her. Before I could speak, a PICU nurse whisked the blind down in his room and his petrified face disappeared from our view.

Abigail was a small girl who had struggled for most of her short life. We knew her and her family well. We had promised Joan, her mother, that if it became clear the end was near we would make sure she was with her daughter.

I have learnt in years of helping parents hold their child as their life ebbs away that mothers and fathers mostly want to be present during resuscitation attempts. It is possible to honour their presence and unique relationship with their child, while at the same time intervening with medications and procedures aimed at reversing the process of dying. Joan walked into the room, swaying with distress.

She howled. She screamed. She shouted her daughter's name. I guided her to sit beside Abigail's head as we continued to work. I murmured soft words to ground her. I told her she could leave with one of the nurses if she wished, or she could stay. She shook her head, 'I'll stay, I'll stay with her,' tears flooding her eyes and nose. We worked for what felt like hours.

Sadness began to soak the atmosphere in the room as it dawned on everyone present that our efforts had not been and would not be successful. Abigail's heart was resolute. It would not beat again. Every possible intervention had been exhausted.

I thanked the team for their efforts, scooped up Abigail and gently placed her in Joan's arms. There are no suitable words to explain these actions, any of which are made intuitively, with tenderness and love. Joan held her small girl for hours. She washed her body, the nurses guiding her hands, and dressed Abigail in white cotton pyjamas. The nurses draw a particular energy around themselves in these moments. It is an energy that is protective, loyal and quiet.

'Johnny is very upset.' His nurse Eden stopped me as I finally left Abigail's room.

My spirit shrivelled as I thought of his terrified face. I went in to him and his father and we sat together and chatted through what he had witnessed from his room. I gave an explanation in simple words, but I knew from the way he was avoiding my gaze that he couldn't listen to me at that time. 'I will come back tomorrow, and we can talk again,' I said.

The following day was Saturday. Weekends can be calmer and sometimes allow a little more time to spend with the families of children in intensive care. We sat together and this time Johnny was a little more forthcoming on what he had seen and how he felt.

I hadn't realised that Johnny and Abigail had met several times before on the ward and in the outpatient clinic. They both had complicated medical issues and had often been together in the playroom on the cardiac ward while waiting for a test or a review. On this admission Abigail had given him a tired wave as she had been admitted. Johnny had had his planned surgery and was on the way to recovery. The difference between them, as he survived, was not lost on the boy who had already seen more in his life than most adults.

On top of everything he was already dealing with, he now questioned why he was the lucky one. Witnessing the death of a child leaves a tattoo on the mind, an image that never leaves, no matter how many years have passed. We didn't want that for Johnny, but it had already happened.

Over the next few days Johnny got stronger, walking with the physiotherapist Gillian around the PICU. He had a little cart on wheels that his chest drains sat on, and he lurched around unsteadily, pulling drips, pumps, pacemaker, monitor and drains along with him. He resembled an explorer, bravely pushing out into the wild sea with his laden ship low in the water. He was pale and tense. Several times I saw him look anxiously at the door into Abigail's room, as if he expected her to wave at him again. But Abigail was now in the mortuary.

And Johnny went home.

Months later, Joan got in touch through Helene, one of the cardiac nurse specialists. 'She wants to ask you something,' said the nurse. 'I tried to find out what it was, but she said she needed to ask you, as you were there when Abigail died.'

I emailed Joan to set up a time to call her. Grieving parents often find it exceptionally difficult to talk on the phone, especially without having time to prepare themselves. I remembered my own self-imposed isolation. Parents dodge the nurses who are trying to follow up with them until they are ready to engage. Putting aside a little time and finding a quiet room to make a call from is the final piece of the jigsaw that makes this important conversation happen.

I rang Joan. We made the obligatory small-talk for a while, settling in to where we needed to be, feeling the edges of each other's company. I wondered as we were chatting when the right moment was to divert into the matter that Joan wanted to explore. I decided to leave it to her – she might have changed her mind and no longer wanted to go there today.

'I hope you don't mind me getting in touch . . .?' she asked.

'Not at all. Although we know each other from the most difficult of situations, it's still a pleasure to hear from you,' I replied, sure now that she had something to tease out, and that she was trying to work up the courage to phrase the next question.

'I have something I can't settle in my mind, and it's bothering me so much ...' Her voice cracked.

'Take your time, Joan,' I said. 'We can take our time with this.'

'Thanks,' she said, her voice tremulous. I stayed silent.

A moment passed.

'I keep asking myself if Abi was scared when – when you were all working on her ... whether she was in pain and frightened ...' Joan trailed off, a sob in the last word.

My mind flipped back to that warm afternoon in the PICU, sun streaming through the windows as Abigail's heart came to a stop. Beads of sweat on the cardiology registrar's forehead as he did compressions on her chest to try to revive her. Looking up and seeing Johnny's terrified face.

'Joan, we made sure that Abigail was asleep. In the minutes before her heart stopped beating, I had checked all the medication infusions she was receiving – two were strong painkillers and sedatives. As we gave more adrenaline doses, we also gave a different, stronger painkiller,' I explained, giving her question weight and focus. 'It's a part of care we take very seriously, Joan,' I continued. 'She was so weak, she needed rest. As her heart slowed, her blood pressure fell, and that would have made Abigail feel sleepy even without the medication. But we don't take a chance on that – it's part of our normal care during such an event. We give a gentle painkiller that also brings sleep.'

It was not the first time I had been asked this question, although I had not encountered a parent who had worried about it for so many months before asking. It made me feel physically sick to think of the path she found herself on right now. I scrambled inside to claw back her story and not mingle it with mine. I took a long deliberate breath, said, 'Abigail', in my mind, then aloud, 'Joan, Abi was deeply asleep and didn't have any pain.'

I heard Joan crying quietly, and the distance of the phone call made me ache to see her and do better, do more to salve her wounds. I ended the call, 'You did everything for her, Joan. You held her at the end, just as you held her at the start of her life. You did not fail her in any way. None of this was your fault. It's incredibly important that you know you didn't let her down, ever. You are a wonderful mother.'

It is to these conversations that I bring Beatrice, and all that we lived through, as an ally. Surefooted, with her presence in my heart, she guides my words and tone.

22. Moving Daily

'The strength of a nation derives from the integrity of the home.'

Confucius

We do research projects in the PICU to help us better understand the illnesses of children and young people. It's an aspect of medical care I have always loved. Some healthcare staff enjoy laboratory-based research; others do studies on patterns of illness, on medications or surgeries. Having a question in your mind, discovering that other colleagues share it and devising a way to answer it can be very satisfying. This was aptly described by the physicist Richard Feynman as 'the pleasure of finding things out'.

It is a culture of curiosity that we encourage in paediatrics. There are strict guidelines and rules to govern how research is conducted so that children are not exposed to risk or harm. Increasingly, research questions and the design of studies are informed by what the patients and their families would like to know about.

Because children live in the care of their parents, guardians or the state, the impact of society and social policy is huge on their lives. Like many intensive-care services around the world, we noticed that many of the children admitted were from a home where there were significant financial and/or social challenges. I had seen this clearly when working on the other side of the world, in Melbourne. Ireland was no different.

We mapped the addresses of children on the regional socioeconomic measurements published by Pobal. Children who needed emergency admission to the PICU were far more likely to come from socioeconomic groups 4 and 5. From birth, as a random act of fortune, health outcomes are influenced by where you are born and into which family. This study and results replicate similar studies in almost every developed country and explain why the care of children is political, as well as social, medical and educational.

Being a child living in poverty sets you up for worse health, making it more likely you will need intensive-care treatment. This doesn't feel fair, because it isn't.

Babies and children admitted to the PICU are sometimes described as having 'difficult social circumstances'. That phrase gets under my skin every time I hear it. What are the motives for describing a chaotic or impoverished life with this euphemism? I think it serves to distance us from exactly what it means to live that life, where there isn't enough money to buy nappies or food or turn on the heating. The phrase is used when children are admitted with the electrocardiogram sticky dots still stuck on their chest from a procedure a month ago. Or the toddler with the black teeth, or the infant who has had their surgery postponed twice in the past because their parents can't get childcare so they can't get to the appointments. Like Amy, whom we admitted when she was five months old.

Amy was a beautiful chubby baby, decked out in pink from head to toe. She arrived in the PICU from the emergency department with signs of serious infection. She was struggling to breathe, and her oxygen levels were low. Her mother, Kristy, was with her. It was the middle of winter, and the hospital was heaving with small children who were sick with viral chest infections. In many ways, this is standard winter work for the PICU. Except in Amy, there was one more thing.

When I examined her, I noticed that the skin on her bottom was broken and bleeding. The redness spread across both sides and around to the front. There were blisters in the creases at the top of her thighs. It was all around her nappy area and nowhere else, so it was clearly related to contact with a nappy rather than an overall skin problem.

Her mother quietly observed me as I examined her daughter. As I was working, I asked Janet, the PICU nurse who was with me, to start some fluids and to set up some equipment to rest Amy's breathing. I glanced up at Kristy's face as I finished. She immediately looked down at her feet, in well-worn trainers. There were splashes of mud across the hems of her trouser legs. I said nothing. She looked up, and I saw her eyes fill with tears. She was a young woman, but she was clearly exhausted.

When Amy was settled later, I came back to explain our treatment and answer any questions Kristy might have. She said she didn't have any questions, as she didn't know what to ask.

I said, 'Could I ask you something I've been wondering about?'

She nodded and again dropped her gaze from mine. She knew what was coming.

'Amy has a bad nappy rash. Do you know why?' I tried to choose my words gently.

With some hesitation, Kristy told me she knew Amy's nappy needed frequent changing and that she wanted to do so. But it was often not possible as they were walking around the streets all day, waiting until it was OK to return to the bed-and-breakfast accommodation or hostel where they were staying. She said she felt safer walking around outside.

'Nappies are so expensive, you know,' she finished, with a note of resignation or disappointment in her voice.

My eye was caught by Kristy's admission details on the medical chart. Where the patient's address was recorded, it said 'Hostel accommodation, moving daily'.

Kristy and Amy were supported by our social-work team and nursing staff. Amy made a strong recovery and enchanted everyone with her smiles, before they left the PICU for some time on the ward.

What became of that little family of two, blown along like leaves in the wind, and all the Amys we do not see?

23. He Will Sing Now

'Play gives children a chance to practise what they are learning.'

Fred Rogers

There is great camaraderie in the intensive-care unit. It can be terrific fun, which surprises people who don't work there. Lifelong friendships are forged over many shifts, where we see each other vulnerable and proud, in different measures and on different days.

Families do not see the bond between staff, who work in teams, boosting each other on long shifts and listening to each other's worries. We collectively recall the thousands of children who have touched our hearts, with the funny things they said, the songs they loved and the way they struggled to live. Those struggles can arise from the most mundane illnesses, like a scald from a kettle, a flu or a fall. It can be difficult to make sense of. As with Mikey.

Mikey had the worst case of chickenpox any of us had ever seen. He arrived on a trolley from another hospital, with a medical transport team who had patched him

together as best as they could. We were told the history
of younger brothers with chickenpox and the days of fever
before he arrived. His body looked as if it had been splashed
with boiling oil. It was angry and clearly painful. There
were blisters everywhere. More importantly, some of them
had become infected and he had a serious bloodstream
contamination, which was causing all his organs to stop
working.

We worked carefully through a plan of organ support
and antibiotic treatment. I sat with Mikey's mother, Marise,
to explain the worrying situation. At the end of our discussion, Marise showed me a video on her phone of Mikey
singing at a birthday party the week before. 'He loves
singing,' she said, in tears. Another short video made that
day showed him with a massive grin on his face as he
dipped marshmallows into a chocolate fountain. 'There was
chocolate everywhere by the end, even in his hair,' she said.
'And I gave out to him,' she continued sadly. 'Oh, God, I
can't believe that.'

Marise asked for hope. His nurse and I said we would
do everything we could as a team. We reassured her there
were lots of small things to focus on and to be hopeful
about. Those small things were very tiny indeed. We had
to move quickly and have luck on our side.

Mikey's kidneys were no longer clearing his blood, and
he had become hugely swollen with all the fluid he needed.
He required dialysis but for several reasons it was technically challenging in Mikey to get enough flow through the
dialysis machine. Setting up the pump and tubing is a
skilled task carried out by trained nurses in the PICU. It's

time-consuming. Keeping the circuit up and running so that the clearance of water and other toxins from the blood occurs efficiently is a very specialised nursing job.

Mikey's immune system was causing havoc with his clotting system, and in combination with low flow, the dialysis machine kept clotting off. Although it was tedious to repeatedly have to stop and prepare another dialysis circuit, the nurses caring for Mikey did so without grumbling.

Lisa, our nurse educator who also pulls nursing shifts running dialysis, said, 'If he needs it, he gets it,' with the resolute air of one who gives her best to each child.

Each of the support measures bought Mikey time. We supported his heart to pump harder and his wet lungs to open. We rested his brain and kidneys, and we nourished his body. His immune system waged war using the antibiotics as weapons against the bacteria that flooded his body. As the bacterial cells died, they released further toxin into his system, which caused more damage. The war went on for almost a week.

Some of Mikey's skin died and our plastic surgeons brought him to the operating room to cut it away so that it didn't act as a further source of infection. That was a very low day for his parents. 'Is it hopeless now?' Marise implored. 'You will tell us if it's hopeless, won't you?'

The ripples and pools of hope run like a stream that courses throughout the PICU. As we cared for Mikey, we chatted to his mother and father about their little boy, the brothers waiting at home, his grandparents and everything he liked doing. He loved unlovable things like spiders and mud. It's so important for us to know our patients, to make a powerful connection with them. Each is a tiny human, full of potential.

Every day I walked into Mikey's room I was struck by the music playing. Marise had put together a playlist of lullabies, nursery rhymes, songs from movies and pop songs. They played all day, and we often found ourselves singing along with them, then laughing at each other. I sang and the Filipina nurses laughed and told me to stop. When I made a tragic face, they laughed more. Marise was determined that Mikey would hear the songs he knew, and his mother singing, and that somehow in his sleeping brain he would know that she was there and that he was going to be OK.

I went off shift for a week, as it was school half-term, and came back into the PICU half dreading, half hoping there would be news on Mikey. All week, in between chasing and snuggling my own little ones, Mikey and Marise were on my mind. We work as a tight group of doctors who respect each other's recovery space immensely, and when we have time off, we try to ensure there is little work chat or contact unless it is vital. In this situation I was unsure whether no news was good news. I went straight to Mikey's room.

Mikey was sitting up, no longer swollen and disfigured. Instead, he was cute as a button in blue pyjamas, eating yoghurt. It was a most joyful sight. In front of him on the bed were plastic play figures I recognised from Marvel movies and comics. Marise was playing with Mikey, and when she saw me, she threw her arms around me in a tight hug. Mikey showed me the bad guys and the good guys strewn across the blankets. 'They're fighting,' he said.

'I think the goodies are going to win,' I replied.

'I know that,' he whispered back.

Watching children play in hospital is illuminating, as they naturally confront their fears and reach for comfort. In children's hospitals, play therapists help children work through big feelings and thoughts using toys, books, crafts and art. Later that day Mikey was to have his dialysis catheter and urinary catheter removed and go out to the ward. He had completely recovered, except for multiple red dotty scars and small areas of skin loss over his ankles, which now had skin grafts and dressings.

'Before we go, Mikey will sing you a song!' declared Marise.

'Sure, we'd love that,' I replied, 'if Mikey has enough voice and enough puff.' I gave him a wink. 'Rest now, and I'll come back in a bit.'

All packed up and ready for the ward, I went in to say goodbye to this gorgeous child who had waged a battle inside his body that he would likely never know anything about. 'He's ready to sing now,' said Marise. I sat down beside her.

Serious blue eyes fixed on my face, and he opened his mouth to sing. His voice was thin, high and a little gaspy as he sang 'It's a Small World'. It was a song I had sung many times in the car with my children, driving to visit grandparents. I turned and saw his nurse Deirdre hold a tissue to her eyes. 'Oh, Mikey, that was so lovely!' she said.

'Grown-ups sometimes cry when something is really beautiful,' I reassured him, with a wobbly smile.

'I know that,' he said, with a solemn nod.

Children are the best of us. They come from us, but they keep all that is good.

Quite a few years later Marise got in touch to say that she had returned to education now that Mikey had gone to secondary school. She had completed her training as a healthcare assistant and intended to follow on with nursing in the future. 'I've never forgotten what you all did for my boy. Now I'd like to give a bit back,' she wrote in her email.

24. Laughter and Living

'He is a wise man who does not grieve for the things which he has not, but rejoices for those which he has.'

Epictetus

A privilege of working with children is the close connection we make with parents and families. It contributes to the strong sense of belonging that is found in the PICU. Sometimes a family sweeps everyone along in a tide of chaos. The Byrnes were that family. We loved them all. They were madcap characters we got to know over ten years.

During that decade, their middle daughter Anna was admitted to PICU many, many times. She had a rare genetic disease that greatly impacted on her overall health, including the strength of her immune system. Each time she needed admission she would stay for weeks. And there would be drama.

Her mother, Lou, would call the unit to tell us that Anna was getting sick again, usually with a new chest infection. And then she'd ring from the emergency department to let us know that Anna needed to be assessed. There were no rules or referral pathways that stuck to how this messy family interacted with us. Once Anna was back in the PICU, we'd be brought up to speed on the latest chapter in their lives. Who was getting married, who was having a baby. Which son was in Lou's bad books this week. Lou would often say things like 'You know us!' or 'We're real normal, we are' before continuing with something surprising or totally out of the ordinary.

Humour was always in the room. That humour, with its stream of jokes, tall tales and laughs, bonded us to the family and united everyone in our battle to keep Anna in all our lives.

Anna's father, Joe, worked in a biscuit factory. On quite a few occasions I knew that Anna was back in with us because there were bags of broken biscuits in the tearoom. Broken custard creams happily dipped into cups of tea. They were not wealthy, but they were exceedingly warm-hearted people, who had embraced life with a chronically ill child.

Going home in the evenings, Joe and Lou without fail would ask the nursing shift leader if any of the nurses needed a lift home in their direction. This was their normality. It is not a cliché to say that we never heard a complaint from them about the way Anna changed their lives. They adored her and maintained adamantly that the family would have scattered to the four winds without her fixing them in place. The story they had built around the family gave Anna her unique role as the keystone in the arch.

They had their low moments, too, naturally. Occasionally, in a blend of motherly love and frustration, Lou would wail and grumble about something one of the older children had done. Then she would visibly shake herself, make a self-deprecating joke and resume her sunny optimism.

Over the last twelve months, Anna had hardly been home at all. Between spells with us in the PICU, out on the ward and time in the children's hospice, normality had splintered a little.

'I know what you're going to say, Doc,' said Joe. 'We're not ready yet. I'll tell you when we're ready.'

On the final admission Anna had nothing specific for us to aim our treatments at. No infection, no heart failure. We tried some of the things that had helped in the past. An increase in support, more rest. Anna dwindled. She was asleep all the time, and her colour had faded in the same way a cut rose in a vase loses its hue. An expectant air hung in the room for a couple of days. We knew it was possible that this warm and loving family might need us to carry the burden of saying that perhaps Anna had lived enough. She had lived with grace and seemed peaceful now.

True to their word, Joe and Lou came in early one morning and told the nurses that it was time to say goodbye. They had sat up in their kitchen late into the night talking to all their children, grown-up and small, and had decided that Anna should not linger for them. Joe said plainly, 'She's done everything she could for us. She's done enough now.' He nodded, almost to himself. 'We'll be OK.' The words were said with an air of sorrowful rehearsal. It was clear that this day had always been in their minds, from when Anna was very young.

We had danced around the subject delicately, trying to find the best time and the best words. They were ahead of us, and had grabbed hold of death, that important part of life as they did every other part.

There was a party in Anna's room. Sausage rolls, which had been her favourite, balloons and Damien Rice played loud. Singing along to the music, long into the night. Amid this glorious hubbub, Anna left. Gently.

Getting a glimpse into the strange world of a 'last night' celebration in the intensive-care unit is illuminating. The nurses help with every aspect and encourage families to indulge the interests of the child and their love for them. Music, card games, board games, reading aloud, singing, painting pictures, photography and conversations that go on all night. The occasional dog sneaked in. None of this takes away from the loss. The opposite, I think. It shouts the loss from the top of the mountain, magnifies it and invites everyone who loved the child into it, so that they can share love and support each other. It's not a wake, as the child is alive and at the centre. It's a party.

'God, we'll really miss you all,' I said to Joe.

Lou smiled, tears flowing in rivers down her pink cheeks.

'Yis'll miss the biscuits more like,' Joe said loudly, looking around him.

Everyone giggled, family and staff.

And then they were gone.

And we did miss them terribly.

But they were not really gone, because they joined our stories and continued to shine brightly, a white pebble on a beach, the waves rhythmically washing over everything.

25. No Baby for Her

'Death is not the greatest loss in life. The greatest loss is what dies inside us while we live.'

Norman Cousins

Hospital tearooms have a confessional magic to them. A place to take a break from the busy PICU floor, the operating room or the ward. If they are happy places, a mix of people will sit and chat freely, without hierarchy or grade. On the walls there's a mishmash of staff notices, thank-you cards for wedding presents and posters for upcoming conferences or nights out. The walls absorb lots of stories too.

One day as I sat with a cup of tea, lost in thought, one of my nursing colleagues perched on the edge of an empty chair beside me. 'Can I ask you something?' said Linda. She's a superb nurse, the kind of nurse everyone would love their own child to be nursed by.

It turned out that, although we had worked alongside each other for quite a few years, we had never spoken about her struggle to become a mother.

She spoke now, and I listened. Blood tests, intimate examinations, visits to doctors and clinics, ultrasounds, medications. I was struck that we were a largely female workforce, providing strong and loyal friendship to each person in the team. Yet there was so much we didn't know about each other. We all keep some aspects of life hidden from view, to protect ourselves and others. She had been through experiences that would test the courage and reason of the toughest human. Several cycles of IVF, with its crushing expense and huge emotional cost. Still no baby for her. It is a story we hear often from parents of babies admitted. But, of course, any one of us could be living it, and/or myriad other combinations of relationship or health problems.

I wondered what the question was. It was well outside my limited knowledge of obstetrics and gynaecology. Of that I was certain.

Her question was about the unspoken effects of loss. She wondered about the loss she carried into work each day, the 'failure', as she cruelly phrased it. Did I think it could influence how she did her job, how she cared for parents and their babies? She was very afraid that her continued failure to become pregnant amid other people's children would make her seem distant or, worse, bitter, even cold. Maybe they could already sense this from her and didn't want her with them. Had anyone noticed or commented on a distance between her and her patients? Should she try another cycle? This could be the one to 'fix' her.

She also questioned whether the work she did in paediatric intensive care could be reducing her chances of getting

149

pregnant due to the strong emotions she often had to suppress at work or bring home. Her family had told her she should move out of this area of nursing and look for a less demanding role so that she could concentrate on herself.

These questions tumbled out of the deep, dark corners of her heart. What are the correct answers? I did not know. I do know that significant loss can erode your sense of identity and make you less confident in your ability to do your job. Never becoming the person you thought you would be is a huge loss too, and it is not a pain that is comfortable to speak about. These are the kind of intrusive thoughts that usually jump on your feet and grab your ankles with icy claws in the middle of the night, banishing sleep for good.

We chatted a little more, but what had been said was so weighty, there wasn't anything else left. I told her how wonderful she was, how much we admired her skills and warmth, that we thought of her as the kindest, most competent nurse. We hugged, mentally put on our armour and moved back into work mode.

Much later in that shift, I passed by the cot of the baby Linda was caring for that day. She didn't see me stop to watch her. I saw her saying the baby's name, gently rubbing their little belly, while connecting their tube feed. That simple task was done with such obvious love. A love that would have been clear to anyone.

She lifted her head and saw me. She smiled, giving me a lopsided wink. As I looked into her eyes, I saw how she cherished the patient. And I saw an ocean of pain.

Each staff member carries their own troubles into and out of work. Relationship worries, financial stress, concerns about their own child or parent. It is an essential part of the humanity exchange that occurs within the PICU. Making a powerful connection with a child and their family means glimpsing your own vulnerability. When we put on our scrubs at the start of a shift, we tuck the top into the bottoms and tie them in place firmly, just as we tuck up our personal stresses and strains, still present but out of view.

26. Generosity

'Nothing in life is to be feared, it is only to be understood. Now is the time to understand more, so that we may fear less.'

Marie Curie

Chromosomal abnormalities can be cruel. They are usually utterly random. It is a roll of the dice when the coding information of who we are mixes with the code of another person.

It's not a very romantic view of falling in love and making babies, but it is what happens when our cells marry those of another human, blending magically to make a new one. It is what happened to Barry and me, and billions of couples before and after us. In the genetic mixture that becomes the code for a new human, there may be a little nibble of genetic information missing on one leg of a chromosome or a big chunk added on. If we tested each one of us, we would most likely find tiny errors in our code. Whether these errors translate into an abnormality that can be seen or experienced by a person is another unknown element.

In medicine for children, we see lots of chromosomal abnormalities and the babies and children they manifest in. When several signs are clustered together, it may be called a syndrome. Traditionally eponymous syndromes were named after the doctor who first described the group of signs. The doctors were almost all male and some had connections with beliefs that are now unacceptable. In a move away from calling a condition after the doctor who publishes a description of it, the chromosomal abnormality is used to describe the syndrome, for example in trisomy 18. At the end of the day, it doesn't matter what the genetic abnormality is – the child is at the centre of the frame, and they deserve to be cherished. Their dignity is inherent in their humanity.

Many syndromes are not detected in pregnancy as they don't necessarily cause big structural issues, like heart defects, so their diagnosis is only made after the baby is born and it becomes obvious that there is a problem. This is tough on the parents as their expectations of a bouncing healthy baby are dramatically altered to embrace a child who may face complicated health challenges over their lifetime.

Joseph was one such baby who made a big impact on everyone. He was the first baby and the first grandchild on both sides of his family. His mother, Paula, said that the pregnancy had been easy, and it was only in the last trimester that worries emerged. Joseph stopped growing. Scans showed good flow in the blood vessels between Joseph and his mother's placenta, but his growth had stalled. After some weeks of obstetric observation, he was delivered early.

Even accounting for his early arrival, he was a very low weight. A truly miniature human, and quite beautiful in his tiny form. He had soft black downy hair and long fingers and toes. He came to our PICU for multidisciplinary assessment and had lots of tests to try to assess why and how he might need help. Paula and Stephen, his father, struggled with the endless drip-drip of test results, opinions and plans.

One evening Paula cried, sitting at Joseph's cot, frustrated at how little anything seemed have changed or improved despite weeks in our care. Joseph was not in a stable position to manage without medical equipment, and we were unable to provide reassurance that this would improve. If anything, he was becoming weaker and more dependent than when he was first admitted.

His results came back from the laboratory. Joseph had a genetic abnormality that was severe and exceptionally rare. From the few cases described worldwide, he was not likely to live more than a few weeks, even with intensive-care support. The rapidly worsening weakness we were seeing in Joseph was part of the syndrome and meant he would never cough, swallow or breathe on his own.

We sat down with Paula and Stephen in a quiet room off the PICU and explained our shared worst fears in the light of these test results. It was overwhelming information for them. We took breaks in the discussion, so that Paula could call her mum and dad in, and so they could come back with more questions. It was summer and the room was baking hot. It fitted with the demanding nature of the conversation and all the emotions that naturally went with it.

Stephen was angry that it had taken weeks to make the diagnosis. Paula's father questioned furiously why Joseph had been brought to this hospital if 'there was never any hope'. He felt we had lied to his daughter and son-in-law. We listened and worked our way through their questions as best as we could.

I felt sick leaving the room. The whole episode felt like a failure. Failure to find out what was wrong, failure to fix the problem, failure to make everything right for this lovely family.

The next morning Paula asked to have a word with me. 'We have decided we don't want him struggling to breathe any more. We hate seeing Joseph uncomfortable.'

We talked through what taking away the medical equipment might look like for Joseph and how we could use medication to give him comfort from distress. Paula cried. We called Stephen and he joined her.

'What happens now?'

This is an important question in any discussion of the end of a child's life. When parents ask it, it is often possible to paint a picture in words of the kind of death they might accept and wish for their child. It's a canvas that we paint together, families and staff participating in this important work. It's immensely difficult to contemplate this scene. Sometimes parents have clear ideas about what they don't want, or a thought that is troubling them that needs an answer. I recall a father who had never seen a dead loved one before and was very afraid of this. Almost as a reflex, I remember holding Beatrice as her life ebbed away.

Pain and fear in a child are subjects that must be tackled directly, so that the intensive-care team can prescribe drugs to help with breathlessness and agitation. These are not quick conversations.

'Can you see if Joseph can donate anything, a kidney or something, to help somebody else? Please. If we could do that, it would really help us,' said Stephen.

The generosity of this question took me unawares and I had to suppress a sob as emotion bubbled unbridled through my mind. When parents find the strength in the middle of hurt and sadness to think of another family, it is humbling.

A week or so later Stephen held Joseph close, out on the roof of the PICU. Paula had asked us to bring them to a garden as Joseph had never been outside. We don't have a garden, so Cormac, my colleague, carried Joseph, attached to his critical-care equipment, out onto the roof. Under the starry evening sky, he had his breathing tube removed in his parent's arms and like a butterfly let out of a jar, he was allowed to go free. It was peaceful.

A little later, we took Joseph to the operating room, and he donated the tiny perfect valves from his heart.

After his death and the valve donation, Joseph went home to the cradle and nursery he had never slept in. Paula had described this room with such detail we felt we knew where he was resting, soft yellow walls and white lacy curtains floating in the July breeze.

One of the nurses, Orla, who had spent many hours with this special family went to his funeral and recounted to us how Stephen had spoken of their time in PICU. How the weeks waiting for diagnosis were the gift of time to spend with Joseph, as we supported him with medicines and equipment to keep going for them. 'We weren't ready to say goodbye and he knew that. He waited for us to be ready,' said Stephen.

A simple narrative that honours the beautiful, innocent baby.

Paula and Stephen visited for a bereavement follow-up meeting several months later and told us how much they missed Joseph in their lives. This made me reflect on the fulfilment a parent may take from a child who is simply existing, even though they are not parenting them and present with them in the traditional sense. Parents can accept a changed role with gratitude, especially if they see that they cannot do otherwise.

We looked at photographs with Paula and Stephen and again marvelled at Joseph's glossy black hair and dainty hands. We went through each of the investigative tests again with them both, to provide reassurance that what they had understood at the time of Joesph's stay with us had been correct. We offered information and contact details for some of the brilliant charities that help families who experience the death of a child. It was a sad meeting, and an even sadder parting, as they always are. There really are no words to salve the pain.

Bereavement meetings are all about presence. That's all you need to bring with you – your authentic and human self. These are the days that lead me to go home quietly. To be quiet in the dark of the evening, unable to speak. Instead, I soak up warmth and light from my family, a lotus flower reaching up through the dark water.

Joseph's fragile spiral valves meant so much to the children who received them, used as part of intricate surgical repairs to their hearts. Many would be cared for by the same team who cared for Joseph, although at the time we would be unaware of these lacy patterns of care overlaying each other. Donation can help with making meaning of a life that may have been short. It unites loss with hope.

A gift of love, from baby Joseph.

27. It Is Not Malice

'Fear makes us feel our humanity.'

Benjamin Disraeli

Emotions run high in the PICU, understandably. Families can be boiling with rage when their child is in the unit. Sometimes fury is quite easy to understand, and occasionally it is a struggle to see the cause. There is always a reason at the heart of an emotion so strongly felt and expressed: it may originate in events that occurred years previously. Unspoken tensions between parents or other family members can heighten what is already a testing environment.

When parents are angry, they usually focus on an aspect of medical care: a test result that wasn't explained adequately, a delay in getting into surgery, the long wait for a plan. Of all the emotions expressed in the demanding environment of intensive care, anger is challenging for everyone. Overt intimidation occurs rarely. The commoner situation is the projection of fear and pain onto the staff, who become the enemy. We don't receive specific training on supporting people through anger or surviving when we are the target. It's something we learn over the years.

Many staff cope by putting their heads down and saying nothing in response to aggressive outbursts; others dodge in the other direction. Few take it on directly, mostly because we know we are not seeing families at their best and forgiveness should be extended. That is not always easy or comfortable.

Laurence was admitted from the ward on a Sunday morning. He had a known autoimmune condition but had been stable attending outpatients every few months. A broad, tall boy, I could see that whatever was making him so sick now had not troubled him until recently. That morning, he was drowsy and disoriented. His blood pressure had fallen very low, and his limbs were cold.

His admitting medical consultant came up from the ward with him. Usually cheery and unflappable, she looked desperately anxious. 'I don't understand this at all,' she said. 'His disease has escalated, rocketed, in the last twelve hours.' She tugged at her collar, twisting the fabric, trying to squeeze answers out of it. We discussed a plan, weaving in her immunosuppressive medications with our intensive-care supports. Slightly happier that a path lay ahead, the whole team pulled into action behind Laurence and his family.

I drew John, his father, aside. 'We need to rest Laurence with sleeping medication so that we can fully support all of his organs and give him a strong chance of recovery,' I said. 'I'm very worried about your son.'

'I'll talk to his mother,' John replied.

But Crystal did not want Laurence to sleep. 'No. The Devil will try to take him,' she pleaded. 'Don't do it.'

I sat beside her for a few minutes. Out of the corner of my eye I could see Neil, the PICU registrar, preparing anaesthesia medicines and airway equipment. Two nurses were steadily working to his left, drawing up infusions and priming lines and pumps with fluids. I felt a surge of pride in the team who knew from experience how ill Laurence was and what we would need to do quickly.

Over the last few minutes, Crystal, John and I had talked through Laurence's illness, why he was now in the PICU and why further intervention was necessary. I stood up, anxious to proceed. 'Is that OK?' I asked Crystal.

'No, no, no! I don't want you to take my son. The Lord will save him,' she cried.

'Just go now, Doctor, thank you,' replied John. I looked into his eyes. I believed I saw understanding and agreement there. I nodded and left.

Neil and I anaesthetised Laurence and set up mechanical and pharmacological support of his organ function. The following three hours were calmer and some of his blood tests showed stability, albeit on every available therapy. I called the consultant cardiothoracic surgeon to discuss extracorporeal (heart and lung bypass) support as back-up if any further deterioration occurred. It was a belt-and-braces call: I knew no evidence suggested employing such support in this situation. We always explore and push every possibility when a child's life hangs in the balance.

In the absence of any clear reason why Laurence had precipitously declined we were in a vacuum. My surgical colleague considered the situation, and we went back and forth over a few points before concluding that it was not indicated and would be futile. I was grateful for the kind voice of the surgeon, Jonathan, who always had empathy with any sick child, whether his own patient or not. In my mind another door closed for Laurence.

Crystal and John sat beside Laurence's bed, praying. They had been joined by two of Laurence's aunts. They prayed in a low singsong chant that now and then got a little louder and faster, before drifting down again in cadence. The atmosphere was lulling. Outside the window there was a bright blue sky and the start of cherry blossom on the tree that merrily waved its branches within our view. The room was warm, but Laurence was still cold. His limbs were freezing to the touch, and his core temperature was low. An electrical warming blanket covered his body, and all around him there were tubes and lines of medicines, powerful antibiotics, steroids and drugs to keep his blood pressure up and his heart beating fiercely.

Sunday's afternoon glow faded into evening. Laurence's heart rate dropped suddenly, immediately followed by his blood pressure. His nurse, Roisin, called for help. I was across the other side of the PICU with Neil, making our way around the other patients in the unit. We quickly checked that Laurence's life-support equipment was still in the correct place, that nothing was dislodged or disconnected, while Neil began chest compressions. As Roisin told us the sequence of clinical changes that she had observed,

I examined Laurence's eyes. Both pupils were hugely dilated open, and they did not flicker as I shone a light onto them. I looked up at Neil. 'He's coned, hasn't he?' he said, as a statement really, not a question, as this clinical picture of sudden and terminal brain swelling was clear.

Laurence could not be saved. His autoimmune condition, in tandem with sepsis and other genetic conditions, had created a storm of inflammation, which we hadn't been able to switch off. His family were shouting in the room as we worked. I stood straight and looked at them all. They fell silent as I said, 'I'm so very sorry . . .' Before I could continue, they screamed, 'NO,' as one body, racked with pain.

What followed was distressing for everyone. Neil stopped doing chest compressions. The monitor showed a flat green line, where there should have been electrical activity. John shouted, 'Don't stop! You cannot stop.' He continued to shout this for hours after Laurence's death, furious and then eventually forlorn.

Neil examined Laurence, and as he finished, I softly said, 'Laurence is now dead, at eighteen thirty-five hours. May he rest in peace. We are so sorry we could not help him.'

Roisin reached down to the end of Laurence's bed to switch off the warming blanket. Crystal ran at her, hissing and flapping her hands. Roisin murmured, 'We are so sorry for you all.'

Crystal turned and pointed at me, screaming, 'Here she is! This is evil. Evil is here. Oh, Lord, there is evil here with us.' She groaned. 'She is the Devil. Lord, help us! Save us! Come now, Lord, there is a devil in the room.'

Her sisters joined her, calling loudly on their god to capture me, the evil doctor, and to save Laurence. I realised that I had become the enemy and was inflaming their terror and loss by being there, so I gestured to Neil and Roisin, and we left the room together. Laurence was still connected to the breathing machine, which gave his body a bare semblance of movement, although all signs of colour and life had left his handsome face. It was dreadfully sad and frightening for everyone on the unit who could hear the screaming and desperate outpouring of grief.

The three of us sat outside the room. Roisin put her head into her hands. We listened to Laurence's family praying and shouting. Our nursing shift leader, Shirley, made some phone calls to see if we could get additional support for Laurence's family on a Sunday evening. The following morning was the best anyone could do, and our shared isolation yawned ahead into the night shift.

After a while, Neil stood and left, returning with three cups of tea. 'Are you OK?' he asked me. 'That was quite frightening. I've never seen that kind of thing before.' I was too overwhelmed to reply with more than a grateful nod.

Roisin lifted her head and blew out a sigh. 'In fifteen years here, I've stood in the PICU and heard prayers to more than five different gods, I think,' she said. 'None of them seem to answer. Thanks for the tea. I've to do my paperwork now.' She took her cup off to the side.

I followed her example and busied myself, catching up with documentation, contacting the coroner and pathologist and other medical teams involved. I made a mental note to follow up with Neil later in the week, as he was obviously shaken.

When I returned home late, Dorothea met me in her pyjamas at the door. 'Where were you?' she wailed. 'You were gone all day.'

'I was looking after some very sick children,' I answered, pulling her tight into a hug.

'But, Mummy, I'm sick too,' she said, her eyes brimming with tears. 'See?' She pointed at her knee, which had a fresh graze across it.

'Oh, you poor pet.' I carried her up to bed, as she told me her tale of falling from her scooter in the park while trying to catch the dog. I lay down beside her warm little body and listened to her breathing quieten into sleep. I grasped hard at the comfort my daughter's presence gave me, although she had marked my absence.

My husband came up the stairs quietly to the bedroom where our daughters slept. He silently held out his strong, capable hand. I rolled gently away from my little girl's sleeping form and sat to the edge of the bed. He sat beside me and put his arm around my shoulders. Without a word exchanged, he knew it had been a difficult day. I couldn't even begin to put it into words.

My spirit felt violated, shredded by the outpouring of anger and harsh words. There had been no malice, I knew. It was simply raw human pain.

28. Who Gets the Bed

'Our lives begin to end the day we become silent about things that matter.'

Martin Luther King Jr.

I honestly couldn't bear to see that child's name again on our booking list. There it was, for the third time in as many months. Sam had a complicated medical background and had needed many major bone and joint surgeries. Each had required a staffed PICU bed for his recovery. Last time I had been on 'hot week' for PICU, we had no free bed to allocate for his care, or the week before that. This meant his surgery was postponed. Twice he had come into the hospital fasting early in the morning, ready for a long day ahead. His dad had taken a week off work to stay at home with Sam's brothers, so that Debs, Sam's mum, could sleep in the hospital near him.

Sam was the sun in their solar system: all the plans that must be put in place to make their home life work and for Sam to sit straight and comfortable in his chair. The ortho-paedic surgeon, Jacques, came up to the PICU to ask, please, could we make this happen on the third try. He spoke about how much the planned surgery meant to Sam and his family. He knew that we were aware of this, but he needed to say it aloud again.

We stood at the PICU desk and listened to him speak with such feeling. The unit was heaving with sick children. There had been more than the usual number of emergency admissions overnight. We reassessed the numbers again, like counting the last few coins in your pocket, hoping for more this time. A call came from a ward to review a child urgently. Our hearts fell a little further.

'Just give me an answer, yes or no, and I'll talk to Sam and Debs,' said Jacques, who looked beaten.

We asked for another twenty minutes, to see if we could move another patient out to the ward. I didn't want to rush other sick children out of intensive care, but we were under enormous strain. With a long and possibly difficult surgery ahead, the clock was ticking to keep the operating team on track. Such arduous interventions are often scheduled months in advance to allow external support staff to contribute their skills and sometimes bring in more specialised equipment. Postponing a major surgery had a ripple effect through the lives of the child, their family, other children waiting and the medical teams.

We had already postponed another surgery that morning. That family were on a train back home with their baby, disappointed and maybe – just maybe – a tiny bit relieved not to be living through the big day. The feelings are as complicated as the patients' medical challenges.

I looked at the list of names again. There was Sam, the third booked patient. Even as I read his name, I could see his smile and his vast collection of teddies. The second name on the list was not one we knew from the past. I called their surgeon. They had been listed two months ago, and this was the first available slot on a surgical list.

'I'm sorry but we cannot take your patient today. We're going to do a little fella who's been postponed twice this month.'

There was some grumbling but also an uncomfortable acceptance that somewhere in this unjust situation there was a type of fairness. The surgeon asked about a new date for their patient. It is important to maintain a relationship of trust and the courage to keep waiting, and we always do our best to fulfil a date agreed. But it's not a promise.

Sam had his surgery and did marvellously. He stayed for three days in the PICU, then on the ward for fifteen days and home. His parents didn't know that another family's child was delayed because we made a place for Sam: we would never tell anyone that. And yet on some level I reckon they knew. Families who spend weeks and months in and out of hospitals know a lot more than we believe. They listen to each other, the comments in the coffee shop, the chat on the ward. Body language and experience fill in any blanks in their awareness of all that goes on in the background. Frustration and worry can boil up into angry words from families and teams when we are so stretched. It's incredibly challenging to make decisions or choices around who gets limited resources, manage any conflict arising from them and maintain focus on progressing the medical care of every patient in the unit. We are spinning dozens of plates, and on each one sits a precious child. Every parent of every child expects good care and to take their child home. There are no winners in a choice between giving to one and taking away from another, but we try to keep a positive perspective for fear of straying into the weeds of losing our values.

Debs left an envelope on the desk in the PICU on the day Sam went home. Inside were dozens of brightly coloured bracelets, made with the little plastic beads that our play therapists use to make friendship bracelets with children in hospital. The card said, 'Thank you, everyone in PICU, we'll always be your friends. xxx Sam.'

These patients, these children and their families, do not easily fit into hard choices or productivity metrics. Constantly feeling as if you cannot meet people's basic needs is highly corrosive to your enthusiasm for life as a healthcare professional. Too many of these days sets the stage for moral distress in staff. Our training and education do not cover being unable to provide care when we're working in an environment of consistently unmet needs. It is a particularly concerning situation for staff who have little professional autonomy. You can't change the situation you find yourself in with your patients. Compassion can begin to wane; the personhood of a patient slips out of focus and even basic care may decline. That is the true wolf at the door in healthcare.

29. Take Back Those Words

'Thoughts are the shadows of our feelings, always darker, emptier and simpler.'

Friedrich Nietzsche

Each word we choose can make an enormous difference to our patients. We tend to use phrases with which we have become familiar, which impart a particular meaning. Or so we believe. On occasion, it's possible to use a sentence or a word to describe a worry yet have an unintended effect. With baby Jonathan I got the words wrong.

Jonathan had been in the PICU for a few weeks. He had been referred to us from a neonatal intensive-care unit and had travelled across the city to us in his little Perspex box. We had not been able to accept his care until a bed became available on a Sunday evening. At our signal, the transport team leapt into action and made the precarious trip. It was precarious because Jonathan's lungs did not work.

He had been born almost at term but was very tiny. Unfortunately, his mum Cathy's waters had broken a month earlier and there had been some infection around Jonathan

170

when he had been born. It is not an uncommon situation, but for some reason, which we were not sure about, Jonathan's lungs had been particularly affected by the loss of amniotic fluid and the chronic infection that had followed. A few hours after he arrived in the PICU, Alan, the registrar on duty, called me: 'We can't ventilate him. He's needing very high pressures.'

I was standing in our kitchen in scrubs at 11 p.m., eating fish fingers and making my children's lunchboxes for the following morning. I had been at home for an hour. My husband's mood was frosty: he had spent the last two days parenting our gaggle of small children on his own. I really did not want to go back in. But I knew that this was not a problem that would improve unless I did. 'I'm on my way,' I told the PICU registrar.

I kissed my husband, who didn't say anything. He knew better at this stage. Just as I closed the front door, I heard his voice distantly call, 'I love you.'

Jonathan was a lovely baby. I think when a referral is made on the phone, there are the immediate thoughts and puzzling that occur about what the diagnosis might be, what treatment is likely to help and how we will work as a team to make a child better and get them home. But when they arrive, lots of things change. They become a human. A small person, accompanied by terrified adults. This is where the emotional impact of the referral sinks in. Now we must protect, treat and love his pale skinny limbs, his soft belly, his fragile heart, lungs and brain.

Together, Alan and I changed some of Jonathan's breathing equipment, his medications, and settled him onto a different type of ventilator. He was steadier now, with better oxygen levels. I chatted to his parents, Cathy and Mike. They were unsettled after the move from one hospital to another and were looking for reassurance that everything would be OK.

It wasn't possible to set their minds completely at ease. Honesty is vital in our relationship with any parent. I explained what steps we would take over the next days to investigate why their baby's lungs were so stiff and what might happen. I stopped short of exploring every possibility with them as we were all exhausted, and it would have been difficult to take in much more information. His carbon dioxide level was still a worry but the night passed uneventfully after that.

Over the following two weeks, we carried out many tests. Blood tests, genetic consultation, metabolic screening, X-rays, ultrasounds, chest drains and CT scanning. We gained little information except for what we had known at the start: a horrible bacterial infection had destroyed the minuscule air sacs inside Jonathan's lungs. Just at the precise stage in Cathy's pregnancy when the alveolar cells should have been growing rapidly, like sweet-pea seeds planted in late spring, a nasty *Escherichia coli* had flooded the fertile lung fields with a swamp of corrosive toxin and destruction.

'Would lung transplant be possible?' asked Mike. It's a reasonable question, but transplantation is not technically achievable in a two-kilogram infant. We had no further ways to treat Jonathan, and the longer he stayed on high-pressure ventilation, the more damaged his lungs were becoming. He now required heavy sedation to tolerate the pressure from the ventilator, and his body lay flat and swollen in the incubator.

I sat with Cathy and Mike and one of our clinical nurse specialists. We closed the door and took plenty of time. I explained the situation in which we found ourselves with Jonathan. 'We are worried that at this point we are causing Jonathan suffering,' I finished.

I knew that Cathy and Mike desperately wanted to continue Jonathan's life. It's hardwired into us as parents to want our children to live. That's never in question.

I left the room shortly after to give Cathy and Mike time to think about questions and the next steps. I was not the first PICU consultant to have this conversation with them and I was aware of how draining it is to be reminded by doctors that your child is not recovering. As if any parent needs to be told – they can see the efforts made and they read the body language of each staff member as they come in and out of their baby's room. And yet the words need to be said aloud. It's incredibly painful.

That afternoon, the nurse specialist found me. 'Cathy has made a complaint about what you said about Jonathan. They have gone to discuss it with the patient advocacy team. She's saying you really hurt them.'

My heart sank. I racked my brain, trying to recall what exactly I had said that would have distressed them. 'I don't understand,' I replied to the nurse, who stood anxiously looking at me. I didn't envy her the job of telling me this, and I could see that she'd have preferred to be anywhere else at that moment. However, I knew from the past that tackling the situation immediately was imperative.

The nurse specialist arranged a meeting later that day, and she promised to be there. Cathy and Mike asked that their social worker be present. We all sat together. There was some awkward small-talk while everyone settled into their chairs.

I noticed that Cathy wouldn't meet my eye, and I felt desperately guilty and sad that I had damaged our relationship.

Mike spoke. 'You said we were causing Jonathan suffering. You really hurt us. You know that we only want the best for our child, and it was cruel to say what you said.'

There it was. That is what I had done. I was horrified. I felt a deep flush of shame. Cathy began to cry. Mike looked angry. My mind raced back over the weeks we had known each other, from the very first phone call referring Jonathan to the PICU. I saw me leaving my family late at night to return to the hospital. It was immensely hard not to feel overwhelmed with defensiveness and unfairness. I remained silent for a few moments as I didn't trust myself to speak straight away.

I closed my eyes and visualised Jonathan's fragile form, with tubes and lines all around him. He was their precious baby, the most important thing in their lives. We all knew that he would not survive and go home in Cathy's arms. That was the heart of everything.

'I'm so sorry,' I said. 'I used those words badly and I wish I could take away the pain they caused you. My job is to help you, and I did not help you this morning – I hurt you. I am sorry.'

We talked more, over an hour or so. The atmosphere cleared a little and at the end Mike shook my hand in peace as I said goodnight. Cathy gave me a sad smile. My heart was weighed down, like a box of lead, as I left the hospital and went home in darkness.

In the days that followed, Cathy asked the nurse caring for Jonathan if they could take him out of the incubator and hold him on Saturday. His nurse called me, and I popped in to see them. 'Why Saturday?' I asked.

'It's my birthday,' said Cathy. 'And I'd like to take Jonathan home that day.'

We looked into each other's eyes for a moment. 'I understand,' I said softly.

Early on Saturday morning, Cathy and Mike held Jonathan for the first time since he was born. He slept into death. He was peaceful, as we gently supported him into a natural passing, without noisy ventilators or monitors alarming him. He wore a white knitted christening gown, swaddled in a soft powder blue blanket embroidered around the edges with little rabbits. They reminded me of the rabbits in the book *Guess How Much I Love You* that I had heard Cathy read aloud to Jonathan many times in the weeks before.

Cathy and Mike decided to donate her stored expressed breast milk to other tiny babies who were sick and struggling.

Then Jonathan's courageous protectors – his parents – brought him home to a big family of cousins and friends. They had never met him during those long weeks, when he, his mother and father had shared their fight for his life. Not meeting a new baby before they pass away creates its own grief experience in a circle of family and friends. The pregnancy may have ended weeks or months earlier and there has been no visible baby to experience. It can add to the struggle, as everyone around you grasps to make a connection.

It is no less painful not to have met the baby when they were alive. It's just different.

My family and friends never met my little daughter.

30. Two Polaroid Photographs

'Have the stamina to work on something until it comes right.'

Mary Robinson

As the years passed and our family grew older, I continued to work full-time in the PICU. The rhythm of early-morning breakfasts, frequent late nights and weekends on call punctuated the school year. We breathed out only on holidays, when it was finally possible to relax. Barry took thousands of photos of us when we were away, capturing freckled faces and endless outdoor meals. Those photos are a family treasure trove of memories. Our children grew up with two working parents, crèche, schools, a loyal cleaning lady and a wonderful childminder called Agata. Holidays were a chance to just be us. They were golden weeks when we spent hours reading, swimming, playing board games and cards, singing and telling stories.

Once a holiday was finished, it was back to the daily whirlwind of phone calls, conversations, clinical procedures and teaching younger staff. There is little time for reflection.

Sick children appear in a hurry and often disappear from view just as quickly.

Bobby came up from the country in an ambulance, all blue lights and rush. Newly born, he already had plastic tubes and medication lines to help him live. The consultant who had referred him to the PICU was anxious that the diagnosis the team had made didn't quite fit how sick Bobby was. 'I think this was all going on for a few days before he was born – that would make more sense . . .' he said.

He was correct.

Bobby had a serious medical illness involving his heart, which had been beating weakly for several days before his birth. His mum, Jan, had noticed that he wasn't moving much inside her and had gone into the maternity hospital. Once she had been assessed by a midwife, she found herself in an operating room where Bobby was delivered in a hurry.

We were waiting in the PICU for him to arrive. As we lifted him out of the transport incubator, he was grey and limp. He wasn't breathing, he was gasping. He was clearly a well-grown baby, but he was critically sick now. Over the next few days his heart grew stronger with the assistance of medication. His parents spent hours beside him, watching every number change on the monitor and every facial expression on his nurse's face. The satisfaction of a baby getting better is always there, even for nurses and doctors who have been working in medicine for years. In every child who is helped to get well, there is a sky-is-the-limit feeling of growth and potential. The early hours and days when a wave of improvement washes into what previously appeared very bleak is a wonderful taste of what hopefully lies ahead.

But Bobby began to have seizures. First his nurse noticed some trembling movements of his mouth. Jan was sitting by his bed holding Bobby's hand, and she felt it shake and pull. The seizures continued and stopped when we gave drugs to treat them. It was very worrying. We were afraid that as he was recovering from his heart illness and starting to wake up, we were now seeing a problem with his brain.

The scanner in the radiology department was unavailable for two days due to maintenance so we had to wait to get more information. In the meantime, we did an electrical recording of Bobby's brain activity. It appeared to be extremely abnormal. They were not an easy two days for Jan and Padraig, his parents, with the hours of uncertainty crawling by. The atmosphere at the bed became tense as Padraig asked every hour when the MRI scan would take place.

The MRI scan of Bobby's brain was awful. There were changes throughout every part, all indicating that during the time his heart had been weak, his brain had not received enough blood flow. The parts of the brain that manage our thinking, our movement and our personality had all been affected. One of our gentle, softly spoken neurologists came to see Jan and Padraig. We all sat together in a quiet room, and we explained what Bobby's brain scan showed and what this meant for him. 'His future is very uncertain, even more uncertain than usual. It could be very dark,' we said.

'I will take him home,' said Bobby's mother. She spoke firmly.

I have heard that tone of voice so many times over the years. Those five words carry the understanding and acceptance that goes with a terrible message that has been heard and a will to carry on. In those words, fate is sealed as a mother grasps the reality that perhaps there is no other choice for her to make. Out of this awful situation, Bobby's mother and father found a common purpose, which they simply had to fulfil despite the unknown that lay ahead. Of course, none of us knows what lies ahead in life, but only a few people can see uncertainty so clearly and reach out to embrace it with dignity and love.

Bobby came off all the critical-care support as his heart recovered completely. Our heart, lungs and kidneys are more resilient to damage than our brain. He was pink, and when the nurses washed him, his fluffy skin and hair caught the sunlight, and he looked as if he was tinged with gold. He was a beautiful newborn baby. As Jan brought him down from the ward and into the PICU to say goodbye, it was a muted greeting. Bobby slept in his car seat, snuggled up in a blue knitted hat, blanket and booties. His big brothers were eagerly waiting to meet him for the first time. The unknown nature of what faced the family made the farewell less celebratory than usual.

'Courage,' I whispered to myself under my breath, recalling a French nurse who had once said that word to me, a word of encouragement to a frightened mother.

Three years later I found a letter in my hospital post-box. From Jan. 'You probably don't remember us . . .' she began.

We always do.

'I thought you might like to see some pictures of Bobby playing in the garden with his brothers.'

I hardly dared to look at them. In the envelope, with the letter, were two Polaroid photographs. A photo of a little boy in yellow shorts, playing with a digger. 'Bobby, age 3' was inked on the back. In the second photograph four boys of different sizes were sitting splashing and smiling in a paddling pool. 'Bobby is the ringleader' was written on the back of that one. In her letter, Jan described their family life of pets, school, play and dinners together. 'He still has a weak arm and hand,' she wrote, 'but I work on it every day with him.'

I sat down alone in the post room overwhelmed with sadness for other babies and families not so fortunate, and pure relief and joy for Bobby, who was thriving with the love of his mother and father. They had the strongest will to squeeze the very best out of their situation, and the good fortune to accompany it.

Will and fortune. It very often takes both.

31. Sickness

'As you start to walk on the way, the way appears.'

Rumi

Indira was majestic. She occupies a special place in my heart. She was wheeled up to the PICU wearing a tiara. She refused to be parted from it. On the threshold between toddler and small girl, she was a queen.

This little queen had been in the hospital for several months. She was one of those children people fall in love with, mostly because of her rapidly forming personality, her astounding vocabulary and iron will. She reminded me of my two girls when they were little. The contrast couldn't have been starker between their chubby health and her troubling sickness.

The week Indira spent with us in the PICU was gloriously warm. Each evening after work I took my children swimming in the sea. As they splashed and dived, I floated on my back thinking about Indira. Her diagnosis was dreadful. There had been surgery, and chemotherapy in cycles, periods of sickness, followed by more chemotherapy. The medicines were selected and measured in consultation with international experts, her disease was tracked with tests, and still her prognosis was poor.

Children seem not to recognise the compromise that illness immediately places on them. Grown-ups will tell you what they can't do any more now that they are sick. I think adults mourn the person they were before illness, especially if they believe their health will not return. Children live in the moment of where they are right now and what they are able to do. The fact that Indira had previously scooted down the road to her pre-school, and now could not do that, seemed not to bother her. But if she wanted a carton of apple juice at this moment and you were stopping her, that was a very different matter.

In her room in the PICU there was a box of movies on DVD. Each day I asked her which movie she would watch. We all knew there was only one answer, but the game had to be played. '*Frozen*,' she said, fixing her brown eyes on me with the utmost seriousness.

If she was in good form, I would push the game a little and ask, 'What about *Brave*?'

'NO.' She would shake her head. '*Frozen!*' she would reply, pointing her finger at the box of movies.

One early morning the movie was playing in her room. Her nurse Ann had called me because she was worried about Indira. Something had changed, Ann said, but she couldn't quite put her finger on it. This is always a red flag in the PICU. Because a PICU nurse spends twelve hours observing a patient each shift, they are exquisitely attuned to subtle change. That change is often so minute that words cannot define it.

After I had assessed Indira, I sat to look over her most recent laboratory tests. Her bone marrow was producing not a single cell of any type. After all the intensive treatments, this was an ominous sign. Ann hummed under her breath. Indira gave a sigh. Her mum dozed beside her in a chair. The room felt oppressively warm.

I went out to call her oncologist. When I came back into the room, Indira's nurse Ann was softly singing 'Let It Go' and I couldn't help but join in. Indira tried to reach up and fix her tiara as it slipped down onto her face. Her wasted arms were too weak to move it. Her hair was gone now, just a few wisps above her ears. Her skin had a yellow tint, and her eyes were sunken and dark. Her cheeks were shiny and swollen as she was now receiving large amounts of steroids. She was ravaged with a sickness that only advanced cancer brings. Her parents knew we were at the end but wanted to try once again for a cure. We were all heartbroken for this wonderful family.

With a lot of anxiety, we agreed on a plan to sedate Indira and rest her organs on full intensive-care support while one final medication was tried. I cautiously gave her the medicines to bring anaesthesia and lifted the tiara off the crown of her head. I stopped and looked at it in my hand. Cheap plastic, with peeling silver paint and glued on sparkles. It looked so different in my hand. I'd never seen her without it.

We placed all our equipment where it needed to be to support her, breathing tubes, medication lines and dressings.

As I went to leave the room, I couldn't go any further. Instead, I returned to Indira's sleeping tiny body and placed the tiara back on her head.

'That's better,' murmured Ann. I wasn't sure if she was being sarcastic, but when I turned to look at her, I saw that she was biting her lip to stop the tears coming. We said nothing more.

Indira died that night.

We took comfort from the knowledge that we had loved her so intensely when she was with us, and she had dominated every second of that short time. She had been the centre of everything we did. Ever since, the song 'Let It Go' has brought tears to my eyes. When they were little, my two daughters often sang it in the car, while I swallowed the lump in my throat and stayed quiet. The song disappeared for a bit, until years later I went to my youngest son's show – our rainbow baby Charles was finishing senior infants.

There was a poem about their trip to a petting farm, read out shyly by some small boys. There was a drama routine, which was chaos and had all the parents and teachers laughing. And there were songs. For their proud finale the small children stood with their hands in the air and sang 'Let It Go'. Charles beamed at me.

His earnest face made my heart burst with love. Standing behind him, in my mind, was Indira, the sweet girl in sparkles and a pink plastic tiara.

32. It Is Goodwill

'No one saves us but ourselves. No one can and no one may. We ourselves must walk the path.'

Buddha

We have a working relationship with hospitals outside our country. As we have a relatively small population, with modest numbers of children, there are some specialist services we cannot provide. It may be because we don't have access to equipment or infrastructure, or sufficient skilled staff. Sometimes we have staff who can offer a specialist procedure, but there would be only one case needing it per year, as it might be a very rare illness.

Medical care, like most tasks, gets better with practice. Hospitals that have a larger caseload, doing more procedures, have better outcomes for that reason. If a child comes into our PICU and we feel they need specialist care abroad, the story gets very messy. It can feel as if the relationship we have with other specialist centres is emotional as well as operational: we cling to the hope that they can take our patient quickly and care for them.

Questions boil up as the urgency of a situation increases: where will the care take place? How will the child get there? Which team will travel with them? Who is going to pay? Where do we get an emergency travel permit? Can the parents go too? Of course it always seems to be a bank-holiday weekend when all this kicks off.

It is not a frequent occurrence, which is one of the many reasons why it is challenging. We must also persuade a specialist in another country to listen carefully to the child's story, offer an intervention, accept their care and communicate this decision to their own medical and nursing teams. As it's from one ICU to another, the need is urgent and cannot wait for multiple phone calls or meetings. There is a leap of faith on the side of the accepting team that we are sending a patient who matches what we have told them on the phone. There's a similar leap of trust for us, as we desperately want the doctors and nurses abroad to help the child and send them back to us in a stronger condition. We must believe that they can do what they say they can.

Given that these are high-risk decisions and there isn't usually a plan B, it's extraordinary that the process rests largely on goodwill. The goodwill of strangers. Perhaps goodwill is not the correct word: it's a process that rests on the very best motives that attracted people into healthcare in the first place. It unites the referring and accepting team in a shared struggle for a worthwhile goal. We may meet these expert colleagues at international conferences at some point or we may not. Behind each of the international experts is a large team of trained individuals whose names we will never know. There can be language and cultural differences to navigate also, as we make the emergency referral.

A 'hot' transport of a critically ill child creates a wave of goodness in people drawn into the care of that child.

I have a clear memory of standing in a room in the PICU late on a Saturday night, looking after baby James. Paramedics and ambulance crew stood waiting in the corridor outside for us finally to be ready to move a tiny child from the bed to the transport trolley.

I looked out of the window and realised that in fleeting seconds the long, arduous day had become late night, rainy and black. My mind flitted momentarily to the birthday party we would have at home the next day for my son Arthur, who was turning thirteen. There was no cake yet, as I had hoped to make it that evening. Arthur wouldn't care about a cake when I told him about little James. Far from caring about his party, he would ask only whether the baby would be OK. Our children grew up knowing loss and joy.

A medical team from Sweden had flown over from Stockholm to help us and were going to carry this precious little person to their ICU for treatment. We had done everything possible to avoid this, but now it was the only treatment left. The child's parents had mobilised family and friends to care for their other children. Another family member had a contact in an airline and was chasing down flights. The Department of Foreign Affairs dispatched two people to organise the documents and smooth the path out of Dublin. A garda escort on motorbikes waited at the front door of the hospital.

Not one person complained. No one said, 'I wish I wasn't here.' Quite the opposite, there was a positive and contented atmosphere in the room. Everyone knew that James and his family needed their skills.

One of the ambulance crew pulled me aside as the Swedish team completed their last checks. 'I'm James too,' he said. 'Jim.' He smiled. 'We met before, in Tallaght Hospital, years ago. I was on placement in theatre, doing my paramedic training.'

'Oh, yes, we used to do loads of airway training with you guys,' I replied. 'It was always fun! How have you been since?'

'Ah, grand.' He shrugged. 'I've got a couple of little ones myself now.' He gestured towards the sleeping baby inside the PICU room.

'That makes this work hard, doesn't it?' I said, catching his eye.

'Yes, but it also makes it even more important,' Jim answered, with a wry expression that I could see was skimming over a thousand emotions, a stone skipping across a city pond.

We went on to chat about people we had known in common, where they were now and what they were up to. Working in the health service provides a readymade stream of easy chat and a vast network of friendly faces. People move around quite a bit over long careers, and although there are many goodbye cakes and lunches, it's never really goodbye.

It is worth reflecting on the wave of goodwill that spreads ahead of a little child. If there is karma, this is surely it. Pausing and acknowledging the unending ability of humans to pull together for someone else's child is an important measure of whether we are working within our values. Each one of the large number of staff and family who were out of their homes on a winter's night knew they were there for one reason: to get baby James safely to the care he needed. They knew that the treatment might not work, but they had the courage to join the gamble. It was a shift to be proud of, a shift that made a difference.

And James did well.

33. It Is a Shock

'No man ever steps in the same river twice, for it's not the same river, and he's not the same man.'

Heraclitus

Lots of babies come to us from maternity units because of the complications of prematurity. It is difficult to see other bewildered parents walk the same stony path that my family and I been catapulted along: the struggle of moving hospitals, bonding with a sick baby, expressing milk, keeping family updated and clinging to hope. Each of these was part of our story yet must remain closeted away. The shape of each baby's time in the PICU is as unique as their tiny footprint.

Depending on the length of time that the baby has already spent in neonatal intensive care (NICU), the baby's parents can be in varying states of distress. There are three phases to the psychological adaptation that occurs in mothers and fathers when their child is ill enough to be admitted to the PICU: the period immediately following admission, the period when they are entrenched in the routine of the unit, and the period of recovery when discharge to the ward and home is likely. Recovery can trail into months.

The shock of a baby's early arrival rearranges everything they had previously believed into a different shape. That new and uncomfortable shape can take some time to get used to. Parents may have had little time to contemplate what serious illness will mean for their child and their family.

One night as darkness fell, I saw the father of baby George, whom we had just admitted, walk away from George's PICU cot to look out of the window. I went over and joined him, standing silently beside him. George was three weeks old and had a perforation of his bowel. He was critically ill, and we were waiting for the surgical team to come and operate on him. Outside, I could see the familiar streetlights and the bingo hall opposite. The latter looked busy, with a queue of vehicles waiting to enter the car park.

'Do you see that bus going past there?' the father said to me, after a few minutes.

'Yes.'

'I'm on that bus every day coming past the hospital, and I never knew all that goes on in here.' He was shaking his head a little, in disbelief. Then he straightened up tall, took a deep breath in and walked back over to his baby, who was now sleeping peacefully with the help of sedatives and a ventilator. In front of my eyes, I saw a man bravely and deliberately shift the gears of his life, from the daily commute to the care of his sick son.

I love the children we care for, but I also love working with the parents. They are complicated, emotional and sometimes funny. Each one is a teacher to us.

George recovered and eventually went home.

Now I look out the window as the buses go by and marvel at what people do not know goes on in here.

34. He Is Not Just a List of Problems

'This is love: to fly toward a secret sky, to cause a hundred veils to fall each moment. First to let go of life. Finally, to take a step without feet.'

Rumi

It's strange to articulate that there can be a high, an excitement, when a sick baby first comes in. When I get a phone call referring a child, there is a small dopamine rush. We welcome sick people because we thrive on the joy and satisfaction we gain from helping them get well again. Every new admission holds the intellectual mystery of their diagnosis, the potential surge of validation and contentment as they recover.

Parents of children who are not recovering quickly or who are living with a disability have pointed out to me how we are drawn like moths to the flame of acute illness. And that this means we can unwittingly make others feel we have abandoned those who are not sick enough or well enough. And when they leave the hospital, little attention is offered to them. There may be a charity they can approach for help, or an advocacy group, but mostly they fight on alone. As my knowledge and experience have deepened over the years, I have come to believe that parents caring for children and young people with significant disability are among the wisest and most truly compassionate people you will ever meet.

Angela was mother to a little boy, Patrick. Together, they had struggled all his short life. Patrick was four years old and had a genetic illness for which there was no treatment. His nerves and muscles had steadily wasted away, beginning when he was a baby. As Angela would often say, 'He was born perfect.' Then she would resolutely smile. 'And he's still perfect to me.' She could see far beyond the feeding, movement and breathing problems Patrick faced.

Patrick was in the PICU many times. Angela was proud of her independence in caring for him, with the help of her sister, Naomi, and Naomi's children. Patrick's dad had left them years ago. As a family unit, they received very little help from the state. On one admission, Angela had said bitterly to me, 'I've had to make him palliative. I wasn't ready to make him palliative, do you know?' With tears in her eyes she continued, 'But it's the only service they can offer me, palliative care for Patrick, so I had to take it. But he is not bloody palliative!'

The word 'palliative' is hugely emotive to many parents, and it was doubly cruel that the only community assistance being made available was under that umbrella. Angela knew an enormous amount about Patrick's extremely rare condition, as she had sourced every piece of information available and had lived with the reality of it. She had clear opinions on what helped and what didn't. She was generous with her knowledge and she and Patrick were a feature in clinical examinations for medical students many times. 'I don't enjoy hearing them list all of my Patrick's problems,' she confessed one day, at the end of final medical exams, 'using their harsh medical language. I know he's not just a list of problems; he's a little boy.' Her voice was a little wobbly. 'But I want them students to learn,' she said, with determination, 'and maybe one of them will find a way to help the next Patrick.'

We all knew that a cure was not coming for her Patrick.

On the night Patrick died, the unit was full to the brim of acutely sick children. On the other side of the PICU, we worked as a team to try to stabilise a baby admitted with sepsis. The shift leader, Ger, stepped in behind me and quietly said, 'Angela wants a word when you have a minute. She has a question. But she knows that you're busy.'

'Sure, no problem,' I replied.

In the hours that followed I didn't return to Angela and Patrick as another child in our second PICU deteriorated rapidly and required a lot of intervention.

It was after 4 a.m. before everything began to calm down. I went to get my coat and keys so that I could go home and sleep for a couple of hours. Then I remembered Angela. I stood in darkness at the door of our office in the PICU. I knew that Patrick was comfortable with infusions of pain relief and sedation and that we were prepared for him to slip away into the night when he was ready. We had assured Angela that he was not in pain and was sleeping. But there was a tug of duty to Angela. I dropped my coat back on the chair and went up the corridor into Patrick's room. Angela was lying on his bed beside him, cuddled close around his wasted frame. She ruffled his thin brown hair and smoothed it down again, over and over, caressing his face. 'I'm sorry it took me so long to come back to you,' I said, pulling up a chair and sitting beside them.

'That's OK,' Angela whispered. 'I know how busy and important you are.' I felt a small sting from 'important'. Woman to woman, mother to mother, we both knew what busy and important looks like and how fleeting it can be, to be so cherished and important to another person.

'Can I help you with anything?' I asked her.

'No, it's grand, thanks,' she answered. 'I had a bit of a question earlier, but it doesn't really matter now.' She shrugged mildly.

'Are you sure?' I asked. 'Angela, I'll help in any way I can.'

'I know that, dear,' she said, reaching across and patting my arm. 'You're all wonderful people here, and I'm so grateful for everything you've all done for Patrick.' She paused. 'I know there are other children here who will do better than mine. I notice things, you know? I've always noticed things.' She lapsed into silence. I sat a bit longer with them. These last moments are where the essence of our lives lies. The privilege of being there is never old.

There was peace in the room as Patrick's spirit left. In a sense it felt complete, to let him go, as he had lived a difficult life that did not hold the kind of experiences another four-year-old might have had.

Chatting about Patrick and his wonderful mother the next week with Ger, the same shift leader who had been on that night, I felt Angela's unasked question nag and nip at my conscience. 'I'm not sure I did my best for them that night,' I said to Ger.

He looked at me. 'Why do you say that?' he asked.

'We were distracted by the new admissions, but they needed my time too . . .' I trailed off miserably.

'It's a funny thing,' Ger replied, 'Patrick's nurse that night felt the same. She said it to me the next morning before she left.' He put his arm around my shoulders and gave me a hug. 'We do our best, Suzanne. There are some things that can't be fixed.'

My conscience told me that by stepping away to the care of another, I had not shown Angela and Patrick, in their last hours together, how much we cared for them. We will never know her question, or whether we could have answered it with the words she needed and with compassion. In truth, I felt I had abandoned them. Without thinking about it, I answered the more demanding, strange yet enthralling lure of the small sick baby who had their life stretching ahead of them. Is that even a choice anyone could ever make?

Abandonment is something no one should experience, especially any patient who is coming towards the end of their life. The uniqueness of each individual means that a human life never ceases to have significance, and in medicine this singularity must always be seen. If not seen, it must be searched for, without exception. That is humanity at the end.

35. I Will Blame You

'What's past is prologue.'

William Shakespeare

Bringing up children is the hardest job there is. There are the worries about sleeping, eating and talking when they are small. These become different worries when they are old enough to go out of the door to school, or start coming home late at night.

One Wednesday in the middle of the school year, I had a brief taste of the mortal dread that happens when your child is injured. Arthur was by now a well-grown teenager who played a lot of sports. Busy on the PICU, I left my mobile phone in the office for a couple of hours. When I picked it up, I saw three missed calls from Arthur's school, two missed calls from his friend's parents and dozens of missed calls and messages from Barry. I broke out in a cold sweat as I frantically rang my husband back.

'It's all OK now,' he said. His tone was dull, so I knew he was mad with me.

Arthur had come down hard on the rugby pitch during a tackle and had sustained a nasty concussion. He was fine by the time I called, but there had been a chaotic period when no one knew if he was unconscious or had other injuries. Hence the rapid-fire phone calls. 'I'm sorry,' I said. 'I was really busy.'

The words that hung between us, unspoken: how come I was uncontactable and busy with other people's children when my own had lain injured on a stone-hard rugby pitch? Barry didn't say those words as he loved me enough to know I was berating myself already.

No parent has made space in their life for the phone call, the collapse or the fall off a horse. We know terrible things happen and just hope they never come to our door.

It is every parent's nightmare to know Max's story. It's a story of a little boy who let himself out of the front door to retrieve a toy from the garden, early one morning. His dad, Will, left the house moments later to head to work in his van.

Will reversed his van into and over Max.

Still half asleep, he wasn't sure what the bump was, so he drove back further, then forwards, dragging Max under the van over the gravel of the driveway. Then he had a sickening thought, jumped out and bent down, laying his eyes on the most horrible sight a parent could ever see.

Max came into the PICU on an ambulance trolley, already sedated and with a breathing tube placed by the doctors in the small emergency department in the local hospital he had first been brought to. They had quickly stitched his scalp, which had a huge tear across it and was still oozing fresh blood into the bandages around it.

We carefully lifted him off the trolley and settled him onto our monitor and ventilator. We set about changing some of his equipment and assessing his injuries. We needed more information, so we planned with our radiology colleagues for Max to be scanned from head to pelvis. On review later in the day, we could see that his major issues were a large tear across his liver, both fractured thigh bones and extensive skin loss on his chest, thighs, back and abdomen from where he had been dragged.

Sitting in the parents' room with Will and Jacqui was heartbreaking. They sat in chairs apart from each other. As we explained Max's injuries and what we would need to do to help them heal, Jacqui sank lower in her chair, sobbing. Will stood up and went to her. 'No! You stupid bastard. You did this to him, do you not know that?' she screamed, pushing his hand away and running from the room. Max's nurse went after her.

I reached over and took Will's hand. 'I'm sorry this has happened to you both,' I said. He started to weep. I felt incredibly sad for him, sitting in dusty carpenter's overalls, crying for all that this meant for his family.

Max needed help to breathe for a few days as he had some broken ribs and his lung collapsed under them. His liver began to heal, and the orthopaedic surgeons placed both of his legs in casts to help the large bones mend. 'He'll be as right as rain,' said the surgeon cheerfully. Those funny little expressions we all use.

Fortunately, Max did not have a brain injury. This was the biggest piece of luck he could have had on the day that the accident occurred. His skin injuries required numerous trips to the operating room with the plastic surgery team, who removed the damage, then carefully draped and stitched grafted skin over the gaps. After the first day or so of worry and shock about how he had been injured, all the medical and surgical teams settled comfortably into addressing the issues and focusing on his recovery.

'Jacqui and Will are not doing well,' said Max's nurse Cara, about a week after he had been admitted.

'Have they seen our psychologist?' I asked.

'No, they don't want to,' Cara replied.

When they came in to see Max in the afternoon, my colleague Cathy sat with them. We were occupied with a different child across the unit who had come back from the operating room and needed attention. Cathy sat quietly with that broken and distressed couple all afternoon. I tried to catch her eye at one stage, to see if she needed a break. 'No, thanks,' she mouthed silently. She was joined later by one of our pastoral-care team, June. Together they held the space and listened to the outpouring of grief and anger.

Cathy called me that evening to fill me in on the support she had given and what she felt was needed next: I was going to be in the PICU for the following couple of days. In turn, Cathy drew on my listening ear as she carried the weight of emotions from a devastated couple. We endeavour to sweep up our own emotions in these conversations, checking in on each other, letting each other know that help is there.

About five years later, Will came back to visit with Max and Jacqui. They were pushing a baby boy in a buggy. Max shyly said, 'Hi,' from behind Jacqui's legs. His face had healed perfectly.

Will showed us photographs of them all at home in the garden with their new baby, just a few months earlier. Will nudged Jacqui and said, 'Tell them what you did, love.'

Jacqui blushed a little but went on and hesitantly described several ten-kilometre runs and half-marathons she had completed, raising money for their local children's ward. 'Jesus, maybe we should have done it for ye!' she said, suddenly embarrassed.

'Not at all,' said Aisling, who was shift leader the day they visited. 'Sure, isn't it for kids, for God's sake? Doesn't matter where they are,' she continued, with typically sensible words of reassurance.

There were hugs and thanks from each of them as they turned and left the PICU.

'Five years ago, can you believe it?' said Aisling.

'That must have been a very hard five years,' replied Cathy, with an air of reflection.

'Thank God it seems to be OK for them.'

The impact of serious illness in a child on the relationship between their parents is inestimable, even when the child makes a complete recovery. Trying to keep everything going at home with other children, stay working and financially afloat and not falling into blame and silence is a daily struggle that can have life-changing consequences.

36. What Home Means

'Everyone you will ever meet knows something you don't.'
Bill Nye

Just as working with children forces you to see poverty with stark perspective, patients living in homelessness test the belief that there is a safe place for everyone.

The story of baby Skye is that of a baby born to a mother who had no home. Josie had discovered during pregnancy that there was a major problem with the way Skye was developing. She had already had a miscarriage that year, and the news was a harsh blow on an already fragile person. Josie lived mostly in a hostel, and sometimes on the streets.

We met Skye and Josie, and Skye's father Ed, when Skye came across to the PICU from the maternity unit. There had been some hope that she would be strong enough not to require admission to intensive care, but within minutes of birth it was clear that she needed our help to breathe. We also hoped we would have a few days to carry out a detailed assessment of her organ anatomy and function, before making a treatment plan. But Skye had a problem with her bowel that needed surgery straight away. From then on, it felt as if we were always chasing from behind.

Ed talked a lot with everyone who came to see his baby and seemed to settle in quite quickly to life in the PICU. Josie, on the other hand, always appeared terrified. She rarely spoke and when asked for questions she might have about her baby, she would say, 'I know it isn't good, and I never get any luck anyway.' All parents are offered the support of a psychologist and a social worker when their child is in intensive care, but I don't think anyone was convinced that Josie was trusting and confiding in either of these great professionals. It's sad to see another person so obviously suffering in the moment, but who also seems to carry the burden of many, many previous battles.

Josie had been homeless for several years, staying with friends here and there, interspersed with some time on the street and more recently in hostel accommodation. She had grown up in three different foster homes. The last fostering arrangement had ended when she turned eighteen. Since then, Josie had struggled to make a place for herself in the world.

When she had discovered she was pregnant the previous year, she had been moved up the housing list in the county where she lived. Then she had a late miscarriage, and her application drifted. Within a few months Josie was pregnant with Skye, and this time she and Ed had been given a house to live in during the last trimester. Josie connected a home with having her baby girl. But she also fretted that the home they were given was only because she was having a baby – and that baby, Skye, was now very ill.

Josie never lost her scared, guarded look while she was with us. She would sit bolt upright beside the cot, jigging her leg nervously, eyes wild at every alarm that rang. It was as if she could not accept that we were there to look after her and her baby. She believed that the care would be taken away at any moment. Because that was what she had known before. She was only a year or so older than my eldest daughter, Estella, and my heart tore for all she had already lived through.

Skye's case was discussed at a multidisciplinary meeting to plan treatment possibilities. There was only one intervention that might give her a chance. In the quiet family room across from the PICU, we discussed the possible surgery and the very real risk that it would not work.

'We'll take it,' said Ed.

'Yes,' said Josie. 'We have to take it.'

Skye had a procedure to open a connection inside her lungs and heart to improve blood flow to her lungs. It was a difficult surgery and took several hours longer than expected.

It did not work.

Over the following few days Skye struggled more and more, even on our intensive-care support of machines and medication. She could not be allowed to be awake at all or she had spells of serious instability. We were anxious that she would die suddenly during one of these events, possibly when Josie and Ed were not present.

It was time to have a long and honest talk about the end

of Skye's short life. But Ed had disappeared. Josie seemed unsurprised and even resigned to it. 'Ah, he finds it hard sometimes. He'll be back.'

We tried to hang on to Skye until Ed returned. Her appearance deteriorated and everyone on the unit was distressed by the effects of our attempts to maintain stability.

'I know she's dying.' Josie spoke softly. 'I want to take her home.' She looked like a small, frail child herself, sitting beside her baby, surrounded by machines. Her only focus now was getting Skye to the house she had helped Josie move into. 'It will all be for nothing if I don't get her home,' Josie stated, with certainty. Our social worker assured her that she was not going to lose the house when Skye died. From her face, I could see that Josie did not believe her. We weren't sure we could get Skye home alive. Whether she would be there alive, in their home, for any meaningful length of time or quality was another question. We contacted our colleagues who do 'angel trips'.

A small team of an advanced nurse practitioner, a senior PICU doctor and a paramedic crew make up this special group of people who carry out a duty that many would balk at and most don't know exists. They transport a child out of PICU, on full support, and assist with end-of-life nursing and medical care in the child's home. It's unscheduled and done out of utter goodness.

The angel-trip team lead doctor came and assessed Skye. We agreed this would be a challenge. After much discussion with Josie and the PICU team, the crew said yes. It was planned for the following morning, after Josie's GP and the local palliative-care nurse had kindly agreed to take over palliative care in the home.

The next morning, two wonderful things happened. Ed came back. He looked a bit shaken and downtrodden. He cried long and hard when he discovered that Skye was dying and that she was going home that day. They were all going home together that day, but not in the way they had wished for.

The second wonderful thing was that Skye relaxed. I've got no other word to explain how, despite still being on life support, she somehow looked a tiny bit pinker and was a tiny bit less fragile.

Skye went home with Josie and Ed, and in the background a large medical team helped them and held them gently in their embrace for a few days, before Skye died.

Josie stays in my mind, as a reminder of what home is.

My heart burns with a fierce need to protect my children and their children from ever knowing the scourge of home-lessness. The flame scorches with the knowledge that some children do not know when or where they will sleep.

37. Faith and Forgiveness

'This thing of darkness I acknowledge mine.'
William Shakespeare

It might be alarming for people to know how much doctors worry. I worry that even if things go well the result will not meet the needs of the patient, which may have changed. I worry about all the things that could go wrong, most of which I or my colleagues have seen at some point. The more significant possible complications that lurk darkly in the corners of our minds must be discussed openly with patients and their families. There are other, exceedingly rare, complications that remain unsaid. As our patients are critically ill, there are not many choices to be made as, without intervention, death is almost a certainty.

Like every physician, there are practical skills at which I'm adept, honed by years of practice, and a few I'm less sure about. Setting out all my rational and occasionally irrational fears on the what-ifs would only terrify everyone. I'm not sure if this is humility or self-awareness, but fear about what might occur has disturbed many nights' sleep.

Doctors dread complications. But we all encounter them, and they linger for ever after, a sour taste after a meal eaten years before.

All tales can be told from different angles, depending on the details you noticed and what is important to you. I am certain that everyone has a different take on what happened with Brian. Narrative is the lifeblood of PICU. Brian went home thinking and speaking as the child he was before he got sick, but he lost a leg. That's the summary of a resuscitation that went on for hours and shouldn't have worked but did. And the huge consequences for Brian afterwards.

We were called in a hurry to the emergency department. Resuscitation had already been started on a young boy who had collapsed. We joined the team and were brought up to speed on what had happened. A vague illness overnight had preceded his mum Anna bringing him into the hospital just two hours ago. It didn't sound like an illness that would spiral quickly into him collapsing without warning.

We followed our standard plan of medications and actions that guide us in this situation. When a child has a cardiac arrest in a hospital and they have not been sick for long beforehand, the chances of reviving them are reasonably good in the first few minutes. That was our optimistic expectation as we worked together. On this occasion, nothing helped.

The clock on the screen ticked past. We regrouped with blood-test results. We picked over the history of his arrival in the hospital again – working our way through potential causes and trying to fix anything that could be fixed. There was no sign of Brian's heartbeat returning. An ultrasound of his heart showed a picture we so rarely see – a heart that is not moving. Whenever I see a human heart sitting like a stone on the screen, my own heart aches in empathy.

Fifty minutes into the ordeal, I left the room to talk to his mother, who was sitting outside. I saw some shocked staff standing outside the room where we were working. One young nurse was crying. A ripple of shock and grief moves through a small hospital when a child dies suddenly.

I explained to Anna that in the absence of any issue we could find to remedy, and when the resuscitation has gone on so long, we must stop our efforts. 'Please, no, please don't stop,' she wailed. 'Oh, God, bring him back, please.' She tumbled onto her knees on the cold tiled floor. She prayed loudly and I could not interrupt her further. I went back into the room where Brian lay.

'He has a heartbeat,' exclaimed one of the nurses. We quickly felt for a pulse and stared at the monitor. I grabbed a stethoscope and placed the bell over the left side of his thin chest. It was true: after fifty-five minutes, Brian's heart had started beating again.

The most likely cause of such a sudden deterioration is overwhelming infection. Brian had received antibiotics much earlier, but we continued to chase and worry about this possibility. We took him up to the PICU. It was early evening. Over the following night he had four further short cardiac arrests, and each time he came back weakly. I did not think he would survive until dawn, and again I sat with Anna to tell her this. Again, she prayed. She told me that God had brought him back for a reason and only God would take him away. She asked me to pause for a minute and pray with her. I closed my eyes and listened to her pleading for God to intervene. I could find no prayer of my own.

Due to difficulty in placing a special dialysis catheter in a blood vessel at the top of Brian's leg during efforts to keep him alive, he lost blood flow to it. That was a major problem. When we somehow stabilised his condition, a surgeon with skills in the area attended from another hospital. It was now Saturday afternoon. The surgeon answered my phone call and listened carefully. 'I'll pick up some equipment and I'll be there as soon as I can,' she said. I could hear her own small child in the background of the call. She said not a word of protest at being asked as a favour to help Brian.

I met her in the car park and brought her in with the box of kit she had collected from her own hospital. As we walked up to the PICU she told me she had never worked in this hospital before. I was blown away by her generosity and calm acceptance of the challenge that had been put in front of her. With the assistance of a super anaesthesiologist, the surgeon took Brian to the operating room and repaired the damaged vessel. A lot of damage had been done to his leg already by not having any blood flow. The surgery was against the odds in every way – surgery when a patient has had a long cardiac arrest in the hours before carries a high risk of death. We all knew this, and it weighed heavily on the team.

Once again, we explained the risks to Anna and that she should prepare herself for the worst possible outcome. Once again, she bowed her head and prayed. I envied her unwavering faith in God, no matter what catastrophe was unfolding.

Brian beat the odds. He woke up perfect. He recognised his mother and smiled. His kidneys started working, his liver recovered. His leg did not. He stayed with us for about six weeks, each day getting stronger. His smile brightened every day. His mother relaxed and laughed with the staff as they went about their work in the unit. He was a child who genuinely added to the life of the ward while he was there, and everyone celebrated his astounding recovery from an impossibly long cardiac arrest.

I cannot say why, but that his leg did not recover upset me terribly. Perhaps it was because I had accidentally damaged the blood supply to his leg muscles as I inserted the dialysis catheter in the middle of the emergency. Perhaps it was a foolish egotistical desire to restore every single part of him. Complications are difficult to face, as a patient who has experienced one and as a doctor who has caused it. I see Brian's smile easily in my memory, and I see his withered leg. A warm summer's day ruined by an errant cloudburst.

My last conversation with Anna about faith and forgiveness left me humbled in her gentle company. She told me God knew everything. I think she meant that all our actions and Brian's miraculous recovery were entirely in God's hands, that testing us was part of His plan and He would guide us safely onwards. Her grace left a mark on my doubt in a greater power.

38. Forgotten

'Fágann an bás pian nach féidir le haon duine leigheas, fágann grá cuimhne nach féidir a ghabháil.'

Seanfhocal

'Death leaves a heartache no one can heal, love leaves a memory no one can steal.'

Irish proverb

A common fear after the death of a child is that they will be forgotten, that only their very close family will know their name and it may be too painful to say it aloud. Since losing Beatrice, I am more comfortable about asking people if they would like to chat about their loved one who has died.

In the PICU we talk about the babies and children we have cared for. They live on in our stories. We remember their families, their funny quirks, what they said, their kindnesses to us and the beauty of their child. These conversations take place in the coffee room, at the desk and in the changing rooms. Naturally sprinkled references to little people who have passed through our lives and with whom we have had the privilege of sharing a moment. These conversations are not always sad. They glow with gratitude, kindness and, occasionally, some regret.

Fiadh was a chubby baby who was admitted from the far end of the country with a bad lung infection. She was referred to us by a paediatrician who sounded incredibly worried. Over the years this doctor had sent us lots of sick children, and I don't recall ever hearing such fear in their voice.

Fiadh arrived just as we began to hand over patients from the night shift to the day shift, the night staff tired and itching to be gone. We had almost finished our morning meeting to plan the day ahead, when the emergency bell rang, and we ran into Fiadh's room. She was not managing to breathe comfortably or effectively on the lung support she had been started on so we quickly sedated her more and escalated our support. The morning went from there, the team racing to catch up with Fiadh as her condition deteriorated at lightning speed. The situation was tense.

Fiadh's parents had come to the PICU a few hours after she had been transported by ambulance, and they now sat anxiously watching our every move, jumping as monitors alarmed and staff called for assistance.

The PICU nurse educator, Tara, and I brought them out to the office where I explained that Fiadh's lungs were filled with infected fluid and were no longer working sufficiently to bring oxygen to her brain and other organs. One of our cardiac surgeons joined us, and together we explained that

Fiadh needed a heart-lung bypass machine to do the work of her lungs, and that this would involve a surgical procedure in the PICU. Then Fiadh would be transported out of the country for further support. Kitty and Joel were stunned.

'I'm going to leave you for ten minutes with Tara as I need to go to Fiadh,' I said. 'I'll be back to answer your questions.'

Joel reached up to my hand as I stood. 'Please do whatever you need to do for our baby,' he said.

'We are going to do everything possible. We are a big team . . . You are the most important part of that team, and together we're going to fight hard,' I replied.

The following eight hours involved putting Fiadh on a special support called ECMO, which used a pump to divert blood away from her lungs, through an oxygenator, and back to her heart. This is challenging in the operating room when preparing for surgery on a heart. It's even more challenging when a tiny patient's organs are shutting down and it's not safe to move to the operating room. Behind the scenes, a team of specialists from Sweden were requested to accept PICU care and transport. This meant dozens of phone calls, filling out forms and communicating with everyone from laboratory scientists to social workers.

Almost exactly twelve hours after Fiadh had arrived, she left the PICU. As she had been with us for just the length of one shift, not many of our staff had met her and her parents. But we fretted about her and wished she could have stayed with us.

Several weeks later the public-health nurse for Kitty and Joel's local area contacted us to give us the sad news that

Fiadh had died from complications when she was being treated abroad. It was a huge blow. We mourned the gorgeous girl and empathised with her parents in the fear and distress they had experienced over those weeks.

A few years later, a fat parcel was delivered to the PICU, marked for my attention. I imagined it was paperwork that awaited completion or medical notes that required review. It was not documents. Inside the parcel I found a box of soft clothing, knitted hats, booties and mittens in all colours and sizes. The card read, 'My daughter told me you always need mittens and hats. Thank you for trying to help baby Fiadh.' It was signed with a signature that might have said 'Kathleen'. No surname, no return address. The bonnets and booties continue to arrive. Coming up to St Patrick's Day there is usually an envelope with hats striped in green, white and orange, and at Christmas there are red and white hats with tiny pompoms. Loss is not forgotten. Somewhere, a granny knits and grieves.

39. There Is Power in Books

'Storytelling reveals meaning without committing the error of defining it.'

Hannah Arendt

Babies love books. When I had my first child, Arthur, the public-health nurse gave me a paper bag with three baby books in it at his six-week check. As a young mother, wild-eyed with lack of sleep and breastfeeding struggles, I wondered who was crazier – her or me. 'Read to him,' she said.

'"Read to him," says she,' I would mutter in the middle of trying to get him to sleep or grab a shower. Of course, she was right. I read to him, and it calmed him immeasurably. It calmed me too. Barry and I read hundreds of stories to our children, many of which they can quote verbatim even as adults.

Babies do love books. Any books we had finished with at home, I left in the outpatient department, after one of the nurses working there told me they needed a constant supply. 'No one is going to wrestle a book out of the hands of a toddler in a buggy,' she said wisely. 'Books walk out the door, and I'm not going after them,' she continued, with a wink.

In the PICU we encourage new mothers and fathers to read books to their sick babies. They are often very scared of the technology-laden environment and the terror of what might happen next. The sound of their voice reading to their baby soothes baby and parent. Bonding can be difficult when you can't hold your baby close to you because of equipment and machines. Reading to a sick newborn assists with connection to a baby and a new family who may not feel like theirs. Older children, deeply sedated on life support, also respond positively to the voice of a parent reading to them. The commonest books on the PICU are the traditional *Guess How Much I Love You* and *The Very Hungry Caterpillar*. The staff are word perfect on these.

Maryam was an impressive person who knew the value of books. She was mother to one of our patients and she had such charisma. She did things her own way, reading aloud her law books to her tiny baby, Jasmine, who had been born too early with lots of issues to be worked through.

Maryam was a woman of steely determination. With her brother, she had travelled thousands of miles as a teenager to live in Ireland. The transition had not been easy. It had been a struggle to settle into school, but against the odds she had finished her education and found work in catering. Quietly she had saved her money and plotted a future, starting a course in legal studies. She planned to help other children who were passed around Europe seeking refuge, like parcels of little value. When she spoke about her childhood, we were astounded at all she had experienced. She simply shook her head sadly in response to some questions we asked, which told us how much she and her brother had suffered.

She no longer had her own parents, and honestly described how frightened she was about being a parent when she had little knowledge of how it felt to be parented. She had intended to be 'better', as she put it, before she had a child. Better prepared, better able to parent.

Pregnancy and Jasmine's early delivery had briefly threatened to derail this formidable woman's ambition, but she somehow got back on track. Over the months we watched her sashay regally up the length of the unit, each day carrying a book the size of a brick. There was more than one of these massive tomes. She steadily ploughed through them, her soft voice reading legislation, legal theory and rules aloud to her baby. As Jasmine got stronger, she was able to rest on Maryam's lap, where Maryam would deftly balance book and baby. Each day, she chatted to the nurses, snuggled her baby and read her books. We joked about how we were all getting an education as a result and how Jasmine would be the cleverest child ever born. In truth, we admired Maryam for her powerful drive and vision.

After months in the PICU, Jasmine was ready for the ward. It was hoped she would go home soon after that. I asked Maryam how she would manage her studies with her baby at home. 'My sisters,' she said emphatically.

'I thought you only had your brother here in Ireland,' I replied.

'My sisters are the women who support me.' She smiled, glanced around PICU and continued, 'Each one of you is my sister.'

Jasmine waited in her cot to be moved to the ward. We had done a great job with her. Healthy, bright and glowing, she gurgled and kicked until her socks fell off. With the air of a woman who is satisfied, Maryam picked up her folders of legal notes one last time and left. I admired what she had achieved as a mother in such difficult circumstances.

Maryam passed her exams. We were utterly unsurprised. She sent us a letter with a photograph of her graduation. She stood statuesque and dressed in red, holding her toddler Jasmine in her arms in a matching dress. The surge of pride and energy that went through the PICU the day that photo arrived was fantastic. We may not have been able to remember all the subjects she had read aloud – in fact, I think she would have been disappointed at how little law we had learnt – but we certainly shared her joy and savoured her success. An incredible mother, among many incredible mothers.

40. It Takes Years

'The only true wisdom is in knowing you know nothing.'
Socrates

Looking back, life as a student had felt quite carefree. We studied hard, worked part-time jobs, partied hard and became increasingly absorbed into hospital life. But it is a process of growing, like a plant towards the light. Once you qualify, you jump to the other side of the fence and become teacher and learner. Interns teach medical students, house officers teach interns, and so it goes on. By the time you are appointed a consultant or start practice as a GP, you have been teaching for more than a decade.

Experience with an inspirational teacher can change the direction of a young doctor's life. I chose anaesthesiology and intensive-care medicine because of the people I had met during my training rotations through these specialties. From secondary school to this day, I have been fortunate to meet many teachers who inspired me to remain inquisitive, thirst for learning and be open to change.

Medical students add lots of fun and diversion to the life of the hospital. For many students passing through the hospital on a training rotation, the PICU is like another universe. They usually have a brief visit and a lecture on the reasons for needing admission to the PICU in a teaching room outside the unit. It's the bare taste of a complex and mysterious environment.

Jane came for four weeks because of multiple emails and phone calls. She had pushed and pushed to persuade us to believe her eloquently stated wild enthusiasm for paediatric intensive-care medicine. Prior to Jane, we hadn't taken many students as we thought they were too inexperienced: they might upset a child or their parents, or a student might be distressed by the presence of very sick children. Jane arrived and changed our views. She joined the team and spent every moment in the PICU.

Some medical students focus on the illness as they try to learn large amounts of facts. It takes time and a bit of practice to see the illness superimposed on an individual human, with their personality and special features, and embrace their family in tow behind them. It takes more years to know that the human personality is the most pertinent and enthralling detail of the entire picture. Jane seemed to have arrived in the PICU with that skill already formed. She did the leg work too, though. As I walked through the PICU I would glimpse her in a room chatting to a child's mother, or at a cot helping a baby's nurse change a feeding tube. Or she would be perched on a stool outside a child's room, reading a textbook while waiting for the green light from the nurse to go in. Another day she was attached to our pharmacist Diarmuid who tutored her in medication safety. Our dietician Jessica painstakingly explained the intricacies of nutritional support to her. The whole team welcomed her into the fold and taught her. I think it pulled on the collective memory of being a student, how memorable and important our first teachers are.

We gave her a patient to engage with and study each day; she came back with a meticulous report on clinical findings and the current treatment. Future sick children deserve a doctor like Jane.

Surprisingly, parties are a regular event in the PICU. We have some days of utter heartbreak, so it makes sense to celebrate as much as possible. Birthdays, engagements, new babies, children being discharged after long stays, new jobs – everyone's special days are marked with laughter and cake. As with every other aspect of life on the unit, Jane was in the middle of the parties too. One evening, I saw her sitting at a desk cutting paper streamers to be hung the next day above the cot of a little baby turning a year old. It was an act that summed up the dedication, love and slight eccentricity needed for this work.

The next day we were taking a break and enjoying the fun in the tearoom. My phone rang: an urgent summons to the emergency department. 'Come with me,' I suggested to Jane. She eagerly wiped her mouth of crumbs, and we dashed. In the ED we found a marble white, cold baby, placed carefully by a paramedic on the white paper covering of the trolley, with cold metal rails at the sides. There were other people in the room, absorbed in their tasks. A monitor above the trolley made a loud alarming sound. It felt familiar, yet disturbing. Always upsetting.

The ED doctor was doing chest compressions on the baby. 'We've just started. He's just in,' she said. The paramedic stepped towards the trolley. I hadn't realised she was still in the room. 'His name is Colm. His mum found him not breathing when she came home. He was caught between the back of the sofa and his dad who was sleeping.' In that short sentence, I could visualise the situation and momentarily feel the terror that would have swamped the mother as she found her baby. I thanked the young paramedic for everything she had done.

Jane stood beside me as we did our work. She never said a word, but I was acutely aware of her presence. Now and then I heard her take a breath. I knew she was struggling to manage the scene in front of her. It became clear as the minutes passed that this baby was not coming back to life. I glanced at Jane. Every freckle stood out on her young face, tears on her lashes. Her gaze was fixed on the little body under our hands.

I pulled in a chair, and she sat. We brought in the baby's parents, and they sat down too. They held their baby close and sobbed. We stayed together and quietly absorbed the intense sadness of this moment, the loss of potential, the loss of a tiny person to be loved. I see why a moment of silence is observed to honour the passing of another person – a meaningful mark is made by the absence of words.

In silence, Jane and I returned to the PICU. We walked together up the stairs to our department, people milling around us, going about their day. We did not return to the party.

Later that afternoon, we talked through the event, using medical language to cloak the emotion. I asked her to let me know when she wanted to chat again about what she had experienced that day. She did not come back the next day. She did, however, answer her phone, and we agreed after some discussion that she would take a few days off to relax. I alerted her course coordinator that Jane had experienced her first death and that it had been the death of an infant. She agreed to follow up with her.

Jane came back to the paediatric intensive-care unit, and we were thrilled to see her chatting again to little children and their parents, her shiny stethoscope around her neck and her pockets full of notes. She told me she was as determined as ever to make her career in paediatric intensive care. It was hard not to be touched and smile at such zeal. I wanted her to know that she could benefit other children by reflecting deeply on that loss and by learning the tools to make children well again.

I am certain that that day in the emergency department as a medical student changed her. I know this because I now understand the impact of my own first death. I was not yet a doctor when this occurred. I was a teenage babysitter.

41. Where Is the Doctor?

'I know what it is to be consumed.'

Winston Churchill

It was common for young teenagers to babysit for pocket money in the local area where I grew up. I was fourteen years old and was only interested in hanging out with friends and playing hockey. However, I was already a seasoned babysitter for the children of my family's GP. He had returned with his young family from training abroad and had started to practise in the converted front of his house.

GP practices based in the family home were a good way to get the business started and involve the family as they grew. It's not a popular model anymore, and he later moved into dedicated premises in the town. One Saturday evening, after hounding the small boys off to bed, I had settled down to watch television. The bell rang. And rang and rang. I hurried to the door and opened it. It was a black November night outside. The streetlights shone a distant cold white.

A man and woman pushed past me. They were screaming, but I couldn't make out what they were saying. They ran through the hall and into the kitchen, and I saw then that the man was carrying a bundle of cloth. As he placed it on the kitchen table, I realised it was a baby. A tiny baby, who didn't look real. Maybe it was a doll, I thought. The man's panic and the woman's screaming terrified me. He frantically began pushing on the baby's chest. It was then I understood that they were screaming, 'Where's the doctor?'

I heard the younger boy calling from the top of the stairs. 'It's OK,' I said. 'There's a patient of your dad's here.'

The couple continued shouting for the doctor as they screamed their baby's name over and over, begging her to come back: Alannah. You have not heard screaming until you have heard a parent screaming the name of their dying child.

I stood rooted to the brown-and-white-checked lino floor, watching them. The moment felt faraway, surreal. I saw the kitchen table under the baby. Its varnished pine glowed orange. Above the table was a light, which was pulled low on a spring. The baby lay on her blanket under the golden light. Baby Jesus in the crib flashed into my head.

A tiny dark tear of blood emerged from one of the baby's nostrils as her father continued beating on her chest. There was a crazy jumble of images running through my mind as I desperately sought something, anything, to help. The doctor had told me that if anyone came to the house looking for him in an emergency, I should direct them to the local hospital. I tried to do so with that terrified, sobbing couple, but it was a while before they heard me in the chaos of the moment.

Eventually the man picked up the baby and held it in his arms. He looked broken in a way I'd never seen. The surreal slowly became real. Baby Alannah was dead.

The only other baby I had known was my little sister, and the difference in appearance of this baby even to a fourteen-year-old girl was obvious. She was dead, and I had not been able to help. All trivial teenage worries were shredded. Though I knew nothing of being a parent, as a human I was shaken awake, instantly changed by witnessing their profound loss. Along with failure and fear, I felt connection and empathy, shared distress.

After the couple had gone, I sat down in the kitchen, lost inside my head. A clock I had never noticed before ticked loudly. The air held the shape of the shock. I was afraid to move in case I somehow brought it all back and made it happen again.

Minutes passed. Then I heard footsteps, and a worried little face appeared at the door. I took his hand, and we went upstairs and read stories until he dozed, lying on his side with blond curls falling across his face. I sat for a while watching him breathing, looking at his creamy skin, and noticing that he had blond lashes too. My mind craved every detail of this safe and healthy boy, trying to blot out the awful images in my head, or perhaps to make sense of what had occurred.

The doctor came back with his wife and walked me around the corner to my home. As we strolled through the cold night air, I told him what had happened. He murmured reassurance that there had been nothing else to be done. My parents were in bed as it was late. They always left their bedroom door ajar. I saw my dad sitting up reading and gave him a wave as I went past. Exhausted, I slept well.

The next morning, I dashed down the stairs as my mother shouted it was time to go to Mass with my family. During the service the priest said some prayers for the souls of those who had died recently. He finished by softly saying, 'We pray for the soul of baby Alannah who died last night.' Hearing her name said aloud from the top of the church, I felt as if a boulder had fallen out of the sky and landed on my head. I began to shake all over as tears ran down my face. My concerned mother put her arm around me and ushered me out by the side door. We sat on the stone steps, a freezing wind biting through our coats, and I told her about the evening's events. She was shocked and upset for me, and for the family of the little baby. Cot death was more common in those days, and it was a spectre that haunted every parent. Despite the GP's kind words that I could not have done anything to help those heartbroken people, I didn't quite believe him. We never really spoke about it again at home – that was just how it was back then. Months and years passed, and only occasionally would I allow images from that night to come back to me. That was the die that cast my future.

It was decades later I realised that the image of Alannah has always been traced across my path in medicine. She's one of my own precious jigsaw pieces, lit up in gold. I think about her and the woman she might have become. I think about her parents, too, more than I did at the time she died.

42. We Are Family

'The art of living is more like wrestling than dancing.'
Marcus Aurelius

'Did you see Isabella?' yelled one of my colleagues at me from across the PICU.

We could have admissions flying through the door, phones ringing off the desk and a run over to radiology for a scan all at the same time, but nothing gets us more excited than a child coming back to visit us. We are immensely proud of our graduates and their parents. We are often described by them as their 'family' when they are leaving to go home. Those goodbyes are brimful of emotion, as if we were at an airport departure gate, proudly waving them off with tears in our eyes. Think of the return through the airport arrivals lounge months or years later and you will understand the emotion.

Isabella was a PICU patient from the day she was born, until she was discharged to the ward aged eleven weeks. Three surgeries, two attempts to get her off the ventilator, one brief cardiac arrest, many medications, several hours of multidisciplinary meetings and many of tears and laughter had passed in between.

Isabella had three older sisters. Jen, her mother, had brought in photos of the little girls, like the steps of stairs in age, and we hung them around Isabella's cot. We often do this as it creates a strong bond between the PICU team and the child's family, as we see the connections that surround the baby. Isabella was six weeks old on Mother's Day. My own four children had woken me that morning with oddly buttered toast and madly strong coffee. Barry was in the background, laughing at my expression as I sat up in bed trying to swallow the bitter brew.

After my 'special' breakfast, I hurried into the PICU, just in time to see Luke, Isabella's father, arriving with her three siblings in matching outfits to visit their baby sister. Pale pink dresses with fuchsia bows at the waist and bows in their hair. The nurses teased Luke about his hair-plaiting technique, which he hotly defended. When the girls came in, they were mobbed like celebrities by all the staff. It makes me laugh to see how no one in the world of paediatric medicine gets bored of seeing more children. Toddler brothers, baby sisters, awkward teenagers – we love sibling visits.

Isabella had had a tough couple of days with a new medical issue, and it was a massive boost to see her three sisters crowding around Jen, as she delicately held Isabella on a pillow across her lap. They had brought her one of their story books from home, and Jen read it to all of them. The staff listened too, the scene was so touching. It was a big injection of hope for everyone in the shape of what

Isabella would grow into, look and sound like – if we could just keep going and pushing every possibility to make her well.

In a way it was a turning point, as Isabella seemed to blossom from then on. Families add energy to everything we do in medicine, and their presence cannot be under-estimated in value. In Isabella's roller-coaster start to life, her family's presence around her was the magic medicine she and her mother needed. The staff caring for Isabella needed that inspiration too.

Isabella thrived after Mother's Day. She grew chubby cheeks and dimply legs and put most of her health problems behind her. We had to admit, with a sliver of regret and a bucket of joy, it was time to go. 'We'll come back and visit, all together, as a family,' said Jen and Luke, as they finally left us to spend a week on the ward before making the trip home.

This was a promise we would cherish, but to which we would not, could not hold people. Admission to the PICU is extraordinarily stressful for families. They come back for a visit if they are ready to do so. We were their first family, and we are family to each other with the same loyalty and care.

43. They Could Not Lie Separated

'And ever it has been known that love knows not its own depth until the hour of separation.'

Khalil Gibran

I could add up all the Sundays I have spent standing in the PICU and they would stretch into the sunshine like the Giant Hand of Vyrnwy. In time made up of weeks and months, events that occur on Sundays seem especially memorable, perhaps because we feel our stretched resources most at weekends. The children in the PICU continue to be critically ill all through Saturday and Sunday, but the service does not wrap around that reality. It's an imperfect system.

Initially, the weekend on duty had been tranquil. I had been able to leave the hospital for Saturday afternoon and had made it to my son's football match. Afterwards we had feasted on steaming bowls of his favourite minestrone to warm up. My daughter Estella was secluded upstairs painting, her sister at the movies with friends, and my eldest, Arthur, was working. It was the lull before the storm.

There was a biting wind, and I had lit the stove. Across the city, unknown to the rest of us, baby Grace was getting ready to be born. Grace had a significant lung abnormality, which had been detected on her mother Dee's antenatal ultrasound scan. Her elective delivery was planned for a Monday morning, when all the teams of medical and allied specialists were available. Dee began to have contractions on a Saturday afternoon, two weeks before the planned delivery date. Her obstetric team did what they could to slow the onset of labour, but Grace was otherwise a well-grown infant and Dee had had two previous babies, so labour was always likely to progress.

As Saturday night became early Sunday morning, the neonatologist called me to let me know that Dee was being brought to the operating room for a Caesarean section, as the electronic tracing of the baby's heartbeat was concerning. On delivery, Grace was limp and grey. She was resuscitated by the neonatal team but remained critically ill. The difficult decision was made to place her in a transport incubator to be brought by ambulance to the PICU.

I joined the team in the early hours. The nurses and the bioengineer had set up a vast array of equipment and everyone stood ready to receive Grace. I chatted with Scott, our clinical bioengineer, about classic cars. It was a favourite topic of ours for middle-of-the-night setting up of special-ised ventilators.

Ventilators, pumps and twelve-valve engines.

'They're here,' called one of the nurses from further down the dark corridor.

Scott and I fell silent. The transport team came quickly up the dark passageway to the cot, anxiety on their faces. A second later, we were engrossed in the handover of this precious baby, absorbing information, carrying out assessments and starting different treatments. The hours raced by.

Sarah, our nursing shift leader, called the maternity unit to see if it was possible to move Dee across the city to be with her daughter and husband. Dee was still in recovery and there was anxiety about bleeding so her obstetric team couldn't sanction ambulance transport yet.

The lung abnormality that had been seen so clearly on antenatal scans was much more significant than anticipated. Both lungs were affected, and it had also encroached on the development of Grace's other organs. I called in additional colleagues from different specialties as dawn arrived. They came to the same conclusion: Grace was dying and would die with or without any intervention or treatment that could be offered. We had to change direction towards the goal of comfort and family time. Sarah and I sat with Andy, Grace's father.

We explained everything, then stopped talking.

'That's it?' Andy asked tearfully. 'She's not going to make it? Please?' he begged.

Sarah and I waited with him while he rang Dee. She was anxiously waiting for news, still in the theatre recovery room being monitored closely. Sitting in the PICU conference room, miles away, we could hear her wails of grief on the phone. Andy slumped, whispering, 'I'm sorry, love, I'm sorry,' into the phone. Without saying a word, Sarah put her arms around him as he ended the call.

There was a knock on the meeting-room door, and a nurse put her head around and looked at me. 'We need you to come,' she said.

I quickly went back to Grace's cot. 'Go and get Andy, please,' I told Grace's nurse, Pippa.

Resting my hand softly on Grace's chest and looking at her dainty face and the monitor behind her, I could see her colour was gone. She was leaving, in the swift, senseless way that sometimes happens when a baby grows, is born and dies before the sun has risen or set on their first day.

I hesitated beside her, caught between the thought that I should do more, but not wanting to cause her pain in her last moments. Instead of futile chest compressions, I stroked her body from her face to her feet, completely present in that moment with her.

Andy walked back in with Sarah, and Sarah pulled over a chair. He sat down, and I lifted Grace onto his chest, where he cradled her as her heartbeat faded away. We sat with him. In silence initially, and then after a while we started to talk.

Andy told us about meeting Dee for the first time, how he knew he would marry her. There were funny stories and serious stories. He told us that Dee had stood with him when his father had passed away, even though they had been dating for only a few weeks. The picture he painted was of a warm, generous woman who had always wanted a family around her.

Sarah and I stood up discreetly and left Andy as he called Dee again on the phone. As Sarah pulled the curtain over, we looked at each other, as we heard Andy try to find the words to tell Dee he was holding Grace, and that she had died. Sarah tried again to persuade the maternity unit to transport Dee to her daughter and her husband. It was late Sunday afternoon, and there were clinical worries about Dee travelling and a shortage of midwives to send with her. She had been discharged from recovery and was now on the ward. A midwife would have to stay with Dee to monitor her if she came to our hospital, and it was difficult to free an additional midwife to do this. Sarah was upset coming off the phone. 'It's not right. It's not right that Dee doesn't have her baby with her,' she said. 'There's got to be some way.'

I called the maternity unit. 'I'm going to send Grace over with her father, so that Dee can hold her this evening.'

Sarah came and stood beside me as I gripped the phone. She could see that I was under strain. For an overwhelming moment everything seemed too sad, too pointless. She put her arm around my shoulders as we listened to the stream of reasons why the newly deceased infant Grace should not be transferred out of the PICU to the care of her parents. We stood firm. Grace would not lie separated from her mother.

The nurses set up the cooling mattress in a little travel cot, and we walked Andy down to a taxi. Sarah drew the taxi driver aside and spoke to him. He nodded, then shook his head, turned and patted Andy on the back kindly. 'C'mon, fella,' he said. 'I'll take care of both of you.' Grace's nurse Pippa lifted Grace in her travel cot onto Andy's lap as he sat into the back of an ancient Mazda. I could see Sarah fighting tears. She closed the door and did the Irish bang of the hand on the roof of the car. Pippa went around the other side and hopped in beside him. The taxi took off, and we finally let out a deep breath.

Exhausted, I checked the other patients in the PICU and eventually went home. Before closing my eyes to sleep, I messaged Sarah: *Did everything go OK for Pippa and Andy?*

Yes, all good. That poor mam has her baby with her now, she replied.

We couldn't fix Grace. Her structural abnormality overwhelmed our abilities and medical techniques. Years earlier when I was a registrar training in neurosurgical intensive care, I asked one of the experienced nurses how she could bear the loss of the beautiful boys and men we cared for: they had devastating head injuries from assault and trauma. 'When it becomes clear that we cannot fix them,' she replied thoughtfully, 'I turn my mind towards making their death as good as possible.'

This is a powerful tool I draw on regularly. It is not possible to make all our patients better. It is possible to focus on their death. To allow a natural death. To keep them with their family and ensure that they feel comfortable and loved.

44. You Can Take in Only So Much

'Our deepest fears are like dragons, guarding our deepest treasure.'

Rainer Maria Rilke

Living with a chronic illness is normal life for so many people. My family and I were very fortunate to have good health, despite our loss of Beatrice. This meant that I moved each day from children who were thriving physically, with only the most minor cuts and colds, to children who struggled to gain weight, go to school and flourish. The counterpoint each day was grounding.

I remember being struck forcibly by this one Friday evening. I had left my children that morning as they sleepily got dressed and made their way to the kitchen for breakfast. I spent the day in the operating room, anaesthetising children who had recently been diagnosed with a variety of cancers. They needed sedation and pain relief for a series of invasive tests and the insertion of a special catheter tunnelled under their skin for chemotherapy. One child that day pulled at the very innards of my heart, as he had suffered a relapse and was undergoing all of these procedures for the second time in as many years. His mother looked utterly desolate.

After I had finished in the operating room, I took hand-over from my colleague in the PICU: I was on call for intensive care that night. It was reasonably quiet, and we weren't expecting any more admissions, so I headed home.

As dinner was cooking in the oven, my daughters and I made a cake. We often did this, as it was a good way to distract them from hunger and keep them busy weighing ingredients and licking spoons. That evening, we made vanilla cupcakes, arguing and laughing about whether raisins should go into the mix or not. When the cakes came out of the oven the children grabbed at them, declaring that 'hot cake' was the best kind. The kitchen had a cosy, endlessly happy feel to it.

Then my phone rang. A consultant colleague in another specialty was calling about a girl called Amelia. 'She's going to crash if she doesn't get to intensive care immediately,' he said.

It had been a long and testing few days, with many admissions of sick children. Morale on the unit was low due to a traumatic death earlier in the week. Several nurses had left recently and our doctors in training had all just begun their posts in the PICU. The sick children always take centre stage, but now and then it is obvious that the supporting crew need minding too. But my colleague sounded extremely worried.

I got into my car and headed back into the PICU. Usually, we review patients before we admit them to the unit, but on this occasion his voice and pure hunch made me act more swiftly. Also I vaguely remembered Amelia from past admissions to the PICU, and my memory told me trouble was brewing.

'Bring her down, we're ready,' I said, calling him back, as I drove and thought at the same time.

I walked around the corner as Amelia's bed was pushed into the PICU room by an anxious ward nurse and health-care assistant. One look at Amelia's face and I knew this was serious. If it is possible to be angry, combative and dying at the same time, that was Amelia.

I said hello and moved closer to her, to examine her. Amelia pushed my hand away with a ferocious look. An angry four-year-old is a challenge, even when not sick. Her lips were a dark navy colour, her cheeks grey and purple. The rest of her body was cold and white. It was extraordinary to observe her fight for life – she was fighting against everything and everybody. It was stunning that she could still rage against us even though her death was imminent. A small child who has grown up with chronic illness has a different strength from other children.

Her parents understood why she had been brought to the PICU. I spent a few moments explaining what I was going to do, what the risks were and what they should know if everything did not start to improve quickly. Amelia was their only child, conceived through assisted reproduction, and every step in their life together had been tough.

'We know all this,' said her father. 'We've been through it at least three times before, with each of her surgeries,

241

and afterwards,' he continued. 'Amelia always comes through,' he said emphatically.

When parents tell you they know their child may die over the following hours or minutes, we accept that. But at the same time, it was difficult in this situation not to be unsettled by their stoicism, or their knowing but not believing perhaps. I wasn't sure that they believed what we were telling them, that her death that evening really was a possible and likely outcome. There wasn't enough time to work through this question, which left a worry in my mind. But time was measured in seconds in this medical situation, so that was it.

We started Amelia on a gentle combination of medications, working silently around her as she lay panting and wary. Her eyes never left me as I set up equipment and moved back and forth around her bed. Although her organs were beginning to fail, her mind remained alert. This clinical picture is very different from that of adults who are critically ill: their minds usually slip away at the same time. With children, they stay present, responding to those around them. Each dose of each drug I prepared had the potential to tip the delicate balance in her favour or away from her. The night-shift team were stellar, immediately responding to Amelia's every need.

Amelia's condition improved gradually over the next two days, and she was strong enough to have an intervention, which further helped her. Before she went to the operating room, the anaesthesiologist and I sat with her parents and explained again that there were substantial risks of being under anaesthesia, as Amelia was still critically ill.

As parents, they had heard so much bad news, beginning even before Amelia was born. They had no capacity to hear any more. Her parents serenely thanked us for caring for their little girl and again said, 'She'll come through this. We believe she will live.'

And she did.

Amelia's mum and dad had made their peace with her illness. In a very deliberate fashion, they had accepted everything we'd said over the years but would not allow it to penetrate their approach to daily life with Amelia or dominate their lives. There was very little they could do to change the future. Behind the coping ability they showed, they had accepted quietly that, one day, Amelia would no longer be there. That day, that very last breath she would take, was no longer for discussion. Until that day came, Amelia would get through.

Amelia and others have taught me so much about grief and living with loss. It has been a source of tremendous comfort in managing my personal emotions. I do not speak to parents or colleagues about my daughter Beatrice because it is important that I never tread on their experience, leaning over another family with my own loss, but it has helped me do my work. I have gained so much more from learning to accept my loss by living alongside others who have grieved and who continue to grieve.

There is no right way to mourn. Grief doesn't always happen when you anticipate that it will. It may besiege you even before the loss has occurred. Grief changes shape every day: a grey, nondescript pebble worn smooth, yet enduring.

45. Respite Is a Harbour

'Every painting is a voyage into a sacred harbour.'
Giotto di Bondone

Winter brings challenge to the PICU, trying to balance the demand for more admissions as viruses spread freely through schools and crèches. Many staff working in the PICU are parents too, having to stay at home and care for their own sick children or becoming ill themselves. This adds to the demands of keeping beds open.

In the latter years of his career, my husband Barry travelled abroad a lot. Getting a phone call from the school while in work to come and collect one of our children with a high temperature or a sick tummy was a stress that every parent will recognise, and we experienced it too.

My sisters and mother unfailingly rallied to help, but naturally I felt torn with guilt about being at work on a day like that. Rushing home to check the sick little one was OK, but to collect another child from football practice and attack a pile of laundry inevitably meant that some other job, like finding a costume for a school play or making cookies for a bake sale, would be dropped.

The parents of the children in the PICU face similar juggling feats, and so much more. Those demands can be hidden, as with Siobhan. She had a bad viral chest infection. This is meat and potatoes for us in the PICU. She was a plump eight-month-old who was wheezing and coughing against a tide of viral secretions. It was tiring just looking at her as she chugged along, like a little puffer train.

We had taken a sample from the back of her throat when she first came into the emergency department and the laboratory confirmed the presence of three viruses. One virus, respiratory syncytial virus (RSV), caused havoc in the PICU all around the world each winter, as sick babies flood in for admission and elective cases are postponed.

Oxygen levels in a patient's bloodstream are important. Due to low levels in Siobhan and a lethargic look to her as she lay slumped in her mother Katie's arms, we admitted her to the PICU for mechanical breathing support. When I explained to Katie that this was necessary, her face fell. 'You mean we won't get away with a few nebulisers?' she asked.

'No, I'm very sorry. Siobhan needs the help of our intensive-care equipment to keep her safe while her body fights the infection.'

'OK.' Katie nodded, looking disappointed. 'How long will she be in hospital?'

'That's a really good question,' I replied. 'Most likely one or two weeks, but we'll have to see how the first forty-eight hours go.' We went on to look after Siobhan and I didn't discuss the expected timeframe for recovery again with Katie.

Unfortunately, over the next twenty-four hours, Siobhan became much sicker and required a lot of support to keep her lungs open and functioning. Our lungs and heart work as two pumps in series, so when our lungs struggle and heave, the back pressure on our heart becomes a problem.

As I made my way around the PICU reviewing the patients, Siobhan's nurse for that day, Caroline, signalled to me to come into their room. 'Katie has a couple of questions for you,' she said.

'Grand.' I pulled up a chair beside Katie and sat into it, glad to rest for a few moments.

'I'm just wondering how much longer Siobhan will be here, you know, in the hospital,' Katie said, a look of intense worry on her face.

'Because Siobhan has a nasty lung infection, I think she will be in hospital for another two or possibly three weeks,' I replied. Katie's eyes filled with tears. 'Can we help you with something?' I was trying to figure out where her stress was coming from, other than the obvious issue of her baby being sick in intensive care.

Katie shook her head, stood and left the room.

Caroline looked at me. 'There's something going on.'

'Yes,' I answered. 'Katie appears to be focused on the length of time Siobhan is in hospital . . . Is she worried that she's not going to get better? Perhaps we should see if she wants to bring Siobhan's grandmother in to sit with her, if that would help with the pressure,' I suggested, leaving the situation to Caroline. I had a feeling that Caroline, who was a PICU nurse of many years' experience, would find the best path to take.

The PICU got busier as the day went on, and it was much later before I had a moment to go back to Siobhan. Caroline nabbed me before I went into the room. She had chatted with Katie in the afternoon, and the source of Katie's despair had become apparent. Katie and her partner Rob had another child, Fred. Fred had never been in the PICU or the wards in our hospital but had been a patient in another hospital many times. A teenage boy, he had a severe disability, which compromised his health and left him with a high level of dependency even when he was well.

Katie and Rob cared for Fred at home, with some input from a charity that provided nursing hours. They had not been on a holiday as a couple since Fred was born. Their first holiday, cobbled together with favours from Katie's mum to mind Siobhan, was in ten days' time. Respite care for Fred in a residential facility had been booked months earlier, with further negotiation after his dependency increased in the intervening months. Several times the respite placement had been threatened because the residential centre lost a staff member, and they were not sure if they would have enough staffed beds at the time Katie and Rob needed it.

With Siobhan sick in hospital, Katie was desperately sad that she would have to give up the respite placement and cancel their holiday. But she also felt guilty that she had even contemplated going away for a break and embarrassed to verbalise how disappointing the whole situation was. If only Siobhan had not got sick, or if only it had happened at some other time . . .

Time and again, I have heard mothers beat themselves up with cutting words, berating themselves for all that they feel they could have done, or should not have done. I, too, have lain restlessly in bed at night and made that list in my head of all the ways I failed my child. The cruelty, as the wound turns inward, burns like acid.

It was Sunday evening. Caroline and Ruby, the shift leader, sat with Katie. Rob was at home with Fred. I popped in for a moment and overheard them reassuring her that she was a good mother. That she was making the right choices for her children. Katie seemed to be at the end of her energies, and she gave in to tears. It was a glimpse into the challenging world of a couple caring for their family in the best way they could in the most difficult of circumstances.

Over the following days, Siobhan began to recover from her serious infection, and we were able gradually to reduce the level of assistance she was receiving. In the background, the nursing team worked with the social-work team and the charity that was already involved. Between them, a plan was made to postpone the holiday for a month and Fred's respite care was successfully renegotiated.

'Don't ask,' smiled the social worker. 'I've had to sell another piece of my soul to get this sorted. Sure what else is a soul for, I suppose?'

That comment seemed to sum up our fundamental reason for being there. She picked up her files and left the clinical staff to continue treating Siobhan.

In all of this, Katie had never asked us for anything. A young couple carrying a weight that would break the strongest person alive. Katie had assumed that this chapter in her life was another mountain she would simply have to climb and keep going.

There are many days in life when it is an achievement just to keep going. Families caring for children or adults with additional needs can feel hemmed in, without choices. They keep going but have little input into the services that might be provided. Making choices for ourselves and our family is at the very core of dignity.

46. Grasping at the Reason

'The practice of medicine is an art, not a trade; a calling, not a business; a calling in which your heart will be exercised equally with your head.'

William Osler

What is the word for when you're certain the worst will happen, but you keep going because there's no other choice? I don't know. But I know the circumstances.

One of the emotionally arduous situations we encounter in the PICU is emergency sedation as part of resuscitation. It is emotionally demanding yet it is vital not to allow feelings to cloud your senses or your judgement. Every detail, visual, heard and read, must be interrogated rapidly to make a good decision.

When a child is admitted or deteriorates suddenly, we administer strong pain killers and sedation in starting intensive organ support. It is not possible to insert most equipment into a child's body while they are awake: it would be painful for them, which is not tolerable. If they are 'pre-arrest' or moribund, this is incredibly hazardous.

The bind is total: the child is dying and will die if we do not step in. But by stepping in, they may die just as we attempt to get support started. We may be the last people to speak to the child. I find this so difficult. Sometimes I wonder if I should get used to it. Stop sticking my nose into the mess of recurrent thoughts and feelings, leave them lie instead. Kick leaves over the emotional mess and instead rationalise the actions we take and their almost inevitable consequences. As with Henry.

Henry was a strapping teenager. Until three weeks earlier he had been playing serious amounts of sport. In the last week he'd told his father, Cian, that he was too tired. Too tired to go to school, too tired to go to training. Cian knew there was a problem.

Henry's GP took one look at him and called an ambulance. Blue lights and siren brought him up the motorway and into the hospital. There he was assessed and stabilised. By the following morning a diagnosis had been made. Henry had leukaemia. The oncology team wrapped Henry and Cian in their warm embrace of treatment and care. As part of his chemotherapy regime, he had a special catheter inserted under his skin and into a major blood vein. It was to stay there for a period of months to allow less traumatic infusion of powerful medications and regular blood tests.

The chemotherapy did its work, lancing abnormal cells at speed. Henry's immune system crumbled away under its weight. These medicines necessarily destroy all fast-growing cells. He stayed in protective isolation on the ward.

Cian later described this time as a 'gift'. But that was in retrospect.

The night I was called to see Henry there had been heavy snow in the city. I had walked to work because road conditions were poor. I had a vague hope that either I'd find a trolley in the recovery ward to sleep on overnight, or the snow would melt, and I could get a taxi home, if the PICU quietened down.

It was after midnight. The PICU registrar on duty called me and explained what was worrying him when he reviewed Henry on the ward. I agreed with his observations and went quickly to organise a bed in the PICU. The nursing shift leader Susan went to the ward. The registrar and senior nurse brought Henry up in the lift to us. Cian was with them.

As soon as Henry's bed was pushed around the corner and into the brightly lit PICU room, I could see we were in trouble. Henry was grey. His lips were white. That is how quickly children deteriorate when they are critically ill. His skin across his chest and arms was mottled purple. He was dying. Cian put a hand over his mouth in terror and clenched back a sob. I drew him outside the room as the PICU team started placing probes and sticking dots and a blood-pressure cuff onto Henry.

'Henry is extremely sick. It seems to be a life-threatening infection,' I said to Cian, looking him in the eyes. He nodded. 'We must try to get him on to as much equipment and medication as we can, with as little delay as possible,' I continued. Cian nodded again. I didn't ask him to reply as I could see he was barely hanging on to his thoughts and feelings. 'I must give Henry medicine to make him sleep during this time. But as we do that, he may die as this infection is taking his life away. I'm sorry to say these cruel words to you but it is important that you know the danger your son is in.'

Cian grasped my arm. 'Just try ... please,' he said. The burden of this man's child and their lives together settled across my shoulders, like a strange creature, but oddly familiar.

Cian wanted to stay while we anaesthetised Henry. Looking back, we all knew.

I drew up the medications for sleep and muscle relaxation. I checked Henry's weight again. I checked the correct dose again, saying it clearly in my mind to keep myself grounded. Henry's body would be unable to cope with the correct dose. I halved it. I halved it again. I prepared medication to make his heart beat harder, which I knew we would need.

Turning away from the trolley where I was working, I faced Henry and Cian. In what seemed like minutes, but was seconds, I ran over my collection of anchoring thoughts to stave off emotion.

Why am I here? I began in my head.

I knew the answer. I knew why I was there.

I broke the next three tasks into stages, counting them out as obstacles that we would try to get Henry past safely. I finished by asking the questioning, frightened person inside me to accept the fear that went with these tasks and to move forward into the moment. Choice defines us.

Cian clung to Henry's hand and whispered, 'I love you, son,' as I started to give the medicines to Henry. I said softly, 'Henry, you are wonderful, everything is OK.' I gave him a medicine to make his heart beat stronger, then gave the first sleep medicine. His heart rate dropped. The monitor alarmed. In thirty seconds, Henry's heart rate fell from 150 beats per minute to zero.

We worked on Henry for an hour, trying to bring his heart back to life. Cian stayed beside him. Many colleagues arrived from around the hospital in the middle of the snowy night. But it didn't help Henry. Finally, Cian reached across and put his hand over mine as I stood leaning over Henry's head. 'That's enough now,' he said quietly. 'That's enough. He's gone. I see that he's gone.'

I knew the self-enquiry would play in my head shortly. My personal tribunal as I demanded, in place of judge and jury, to know if I had made the best decision possible, or would another doctor have used superior knowledge, superior judgement, and dragged Henry back from the brink. Doubting and questioning, two sharpened blades we use to refine our abilities. Those razors cut deep.

Henry had a bloodstream infection with a bacterium that destroys cells. The bacteria had somehow entered through the catheter and travelled everywhere in his body over a few hours. He had no immune capacity to fight it. The antibiotics that were given as he had become sick had caused the bacteria to release a toxin or poison as they died. There was no battle, no fight. It was brutal colonisation.

In the hours that followed, Cian told the story of Henry. From his surprise conception to his mother, who had returned to her life on the other side of the world when he was five, to the adventures that Henry and Cian had had together. 'The grumpy teenage years had only just begun,' Cian said, shaking his head. 'I had been kind of dreading those years, but now . . .'

'We're so sorry, Cian,' I said. 'This is so painful, so sad. It's unbearable.'

'Yeah,' he replied, visibly smaller and older. Now a father whose son was dead.

I brought Cian into the Butterfly Room while the nurses washed Henry. I sat for a while with him, watching the light change outside the window. It was a cold light, almost silver, as it bounced off the snow and made its way high up to the window. Cian made some phone calls, and I left, closing the door gently behind me.

Henry looked still. A statue of the running, throwing, jumping boy he had been. For a split second as I looked at his marble-like form, I saw in my mind my daughter. I probed that image further. Then, like a deck of cards spilling out one after the other, I saw all the other children who had died as we had tried to save them, their faces falling in behind one another, their names traced behind them.

We know why we are here. We save many. But not all. A small number of people we cannot help. The mortality in most paediatric intensive-care units in the developed world is less than five per cent. Hidden within that relatively low number are unforgettable children, their families and communities.

Barry somehow knew that it was a horrible night, and as soon as all the children were in school, he drove to the hospital to collect me. When I hopped into the car, I saw he was wearing a woolly ski hat from decades ago. I giggled hysterically, then disintegrated into floods of tears. He held my hand, and I saw his mouth pinch in worry, as he wondered whether any of this life that we were leading made sense.

47. The Voice of Experience

'We are what we believe we are.'

C.S. Lewis

Like every harsh environment, the longer you spend in it, the more normal it starts to feel. The conditions will select those who feel comfortable, like cacti in the desert. That might be true for the staff who have some element of choice about where they work. But parents and their children have no choice. They are the roses in the desert and the reason we are there. We can be guilty of losing sight of how inhospitable the environment is. I've seen the difference comforts from home can make to people when they are adapting to life in the PICU – a pillow, home-cooked food, soft blankets with familiar smells, good coffee. Humans are remarkably resilient and will take a deep breath and endure incredible conditions and sudden change, especially for their child.

That's true for most parents. Frank was a little different, however.

Chloë's father, Frank, came to the PICU having already adapted to intensive care because he had been a patient there many times, from childhood onwards. We did not know this when Chloë was admitted to our unit after major surgery. Frank and his wife Ailbhe waited in the parents' sitting room for her to come over from the operating room. Chloë's surgeon had already been to them to explain what she and her team had done, how it had differed a little from the original plan and why. Unusually, Frank asked for the intensive-care doctor to come and chat with them before Chloë was brought over by her anaesthesiologist. I finished what I was doing and went out to find them.

Frank stood by the window, light falling in around his slim shoulders. Ailbhe sat at the edge of the chair beside him, chewing the edges of her fingers. I introduced myself and sat beside Ailbhe. 'You wanted to talk about Chloë's care over the next few days?' I began.

'No,' Frank said. 'I want to thank you for all you and the ICU team will do for our daughter,' he continued.

I could see these words were important to him, so I just smiled and nodded without speaking as I didn't want to interrupt what he clearly needed to say: understanding what was going on in his mind would be different, I thought, from the more commonly encountered concerns.

'And we wanted you to know our daughter before you meet her, so that you understand how we feel,' he went on.

'That's a wonderful idea,' I said. They sat down on either side of me and played a video of Chloë on their phone. From a photo of an ultrasound scan when she was growing inside Ailbhe, to newborn pictures, Chloë singing 'Baby Shark', then standing at the top of a slide in the playground

and whizzing down to the end to cheers from Frank ...
Images of Chloë tumbled out of that phone. She was there,
a little girl full of personality and spark. Their first and only
child.

Frank then rummaged in a bag, brought out a typed sheet
and handed it to me. On the page was a summary of when
Chloë had become unwell, her symptoms, the tests that
had been done, the diagnosis and the surgery that was
planned. 'I thought this would save you some time reading
her notes,' Frank said solemnly. 'So now you know our
daughter.' He took a deep breath and, as he let it out, he
said again, 'Thank you.'

Ailbhe took a pillow with a pink pillowcase out of a bag.
It had picture of a unicorn on it and the slogan 'livin' the
dream'. 'This is Chloë's,' she said.

'I guessed that,' I replied, smiling.

'Could you put it under her head before she wakes up?'
she continued, her pale face pinched with worry.

'Of course, that's no problem,' I said, as I took the pillow
from her hands and left to go back into the unit.

Chloë had more pain than we'd hoped for that first
evening, and this increased the tension in the room until
we got on top of it, and she slept comfortably.

Ailbhe looked exhausted and went to the parents' accommodation floor to rest. Frank stayed in a chair by Chloë's
bed. It was there that we chatted, and he told me about
his own medical issues. Frank had a genetic condition called
cystic fibrosis, which had first caused problems when he
was about four years old. Over the following twenty-five
years he had been admitted to hospital dozens of times. He

had drains in his chest when his lungs collapsed, he had a blockage in his bowel that needed several surgeries to resolve, and he had become diabetic and would eventually need a liver and pancreas transplant. His whole life had been consumed with treatment and the fight to stay alive. He lifted his shirt and proudly showed the PICU nurse and me his chest and abdomen, which were crisscrossed with scars.

'I am a human battlefield,' he declared, with an ironic smile.

The nurse shook her head and murmured something in the language of the Philippines, before repeating it in English: 'Our Lord has tested you,' she said. 'He has tested you a lot,' she continued, as she gestured with her hand towards Chloë's sleeping form.

'Oh, no,' replied Frank, with a smile, 'quite the opposite. Chloë is my saviour, she really is.' And that seemed to make sense as he stated it – Chloë had given him a new purpose in life, and it meant he had a place to put all his hard-won experience. He knew illness and pain, and he knew recovery.

Frank was determined that Chloë would have a different experience from his. As she grew, she would not face the difficulties he had lived with. She didn't have cystic fibrosis, and the surgery she had just survived meant that she would be unlikely to need PICU admission again. Her story would be different.

The struggle Frank's parents had wrestled with when he was a young boy loomed large in the conversation. They had had to manage their farm and other children, while bringing Frank up and down the country to see doctors.

'You know, all those years, they never complained about it,' he said. 'It's hard to believe, isn't it?'

'I believe it,' I replied, 'because I see that courage and love every day. It is one of the reasons why this is such a wonderful place.'

48. How Happy She Had Been

'Poor is poor, in any language.'

Mary Robinson

Barry and I worked incredibly hard together to keep a strong sense of family. We incorporated our loss into our family's story and Beatrice's brothers and sisters grew up comfortable in asking about her and speculating about what she would have been like.

Their questions came at the oddest of moments. We could be hanging upside-down off monkey bars in the playground or lying on a picnic blanket staring at the sky and someone would ask 'Would Beatrice have been as tall as me?' or 'What songs do you think she liked?' Their place in their little world was certain to them and they were secure enough to explore their imaginations and bring their tiny sister with them. These were surprisingly happy moments for me.

Happiness comes in a kaleidoscope of forms. I saw this with Ashley and Kira.

Kira came from the south of the country. She was four weeks old and had not been home yet. Usually this is a source of disappointment to parents. However, it was a very good thing in the eyes of Ashley, her mother. This was because Kira was most likely not going home with her mother: it was planned that she would go to a foster family. Her older brothers and sisters were in foster care already. Ashley didn't have any of her children living with her. The reasons for this decision were not ours to know, other than that Ashley could visit without restriction.

Kira had been born a little early and had a problem with her heart that would need surgery. She was a gorgeous baby, with thick black curls that spread down a little onto her shoulders, in the way that early babies sometimes have downy hair on their bodies. She was not big enough to have surgery yet but had begun to struggle to breathe on her own. Once we got her established on our intensive-care supporting equipment and medications, she flourished. And so did Ashley. They settled into life in the PICU, and it was a happy time.

Ashley had travelled to the hospital to spend as much time as possible with her child. This was especially poignant as she told the nurses caring for Kira that the social workers in her local area 'had everything arranged to take Kira'. This was later confirmed by our own social worker. There is life outside the PICU, for families and for staff, and none of us ever really knows anything about it. Our lives briefly touch the life of another when we care for them, like the moon passing in front of the sun, changing the light.

There was something about Ashley's fragile spirit, endlessly standing beside her baby's cot, that touched my heart so much. Every morning, she was resolutely upbeat. 'How is Kira today, Ashley?' I would ask.

'She's grand' would come the cheerful reply.

'And how are you?' I'd continue, looking into Ashley's light blue eyes.

'Sure, I'm grand too.' She'd shrug with a shy smile.

She looked older than her years, deep crevices around her stunning eyes, her face lined and her teeth in a poor state. Her state of contentment seemed to grow during those weeks – it was striking. She stayed in hospital accommodation and came each day without fail. Although happy to chat for a bit with the nurses, she often sat for hours staring into space. Daydreaming, perhaps.

One quiet Saturday morning I enquired if the waiting for surgery was becoming too much. 'It can't be great living in hospital accommodation for so long . . . waiting?' I said to her.

'I've lived in far worse,' Ashley replied, 'even spent a bit of time on the street.' She looked down at her hands twisted around each other in her lap, as if she regretted saying anything. It seemed to be more than she was able to share at that time. I pulled up a chair and sat beside her, to give her an opportunity to speak a little more, but she stayed silent.

After five weeks, Kira had her surgery. She was barely the weight to make surgery a possibility, having struggled to grow to the necessary size. It's always difficult for everyone when a patient has been in the PICU for a long time before they go for surgery. It somehow feels like the stakes are higher, which is an emotional response to the relationship that has developed in the weeks while waiting. It's also based in fact too: surgery on patients in intensive care has a lower chance of being successful as the patient, dependent on critical care, is sicker going into it. This was Kira's one and best chance.

It went brilliantly, as did the following few days after. Kira was pinker and stronger almost from the first hour after the operation. Each day after the operation we reduced her support and took away the medicines that had provided the scaffolding to hold her safe while waiting. But there wasn't the same scaffolding holding Ashley. The thing holding Ashley together was being present with Kira.

The day we planned Kira's discharge to the ward, I knew that Ashley had already guessed the plan. I knew because when I said, 'Hi, how are you?' Ashley just looked past me, at the window behind.

'Grand,' she said softly. 'We're doing grand.' She looked as if her thoughts had led her far away. But this time it seemed not to be peaceful daydreaming.

Kira went to the ward, and then to the home of the foster family who had agreed to care for her. Because we knew this was arranged, saying goodbye to Kira felt especially sad. We wished her to be safe and to grow up loved and reach her potential, as we hope for every child. We were sad mostly for Ashley and the loss she was facing. She seemed to have shrunk back into herself and no longer spoke to us. It was hard not to feel we had all let her down ... as she had always expected us to.

More than a year later we heard from our colleagues in the referring hospital that Ashley had died. It was another fragment of a life story, in the same way that the moments we had shared with her were fragments of a much bigger story. The day this news came to us, the sadness in the unit was inescapable. Over a cup of tea, we tried to comfort ourselves by recalling how happy she had been when she and Kira were with us. How we had been a cocoon for them both, as Ashley was held in time and Kira blossomed.

Inevitably, our thoughts went to Kira, her brothers and sisters, who didn't have their mam any more – even though they hadn't had her for years. In those sorrowful musings we included the children who grow up to become Ashley, and all that they suffer in their own fight to live and be happy.

49. Speak the Dreadful Words

'I believe that I am not responsible for the meaningfulness or meaninglessness of life, but that I am responsible for what I do with the life I've got.'

Hermann Hesse

Giving devastating news to parents is part and parcel of our work. Like many things, practice takes the element of distress out of the experience and allows you to focus on giving information clearly and with compassion. Practice cools the temperature of the staff involved – but it's a balance: sufficient comfort in what you are doing to be competent, but not so much exposure that you can't feel what is important. In weeks where we have several deaths, this is not easy.

Rather than a burst of bad news, it is much kinder to ease towards the message, by leading with a gentle hint: 'We're terribly worried about Paul ... He's not responding to any treatment.' Or, in my case, Dr Amolle had said, 'We can see only a dark future for Beatrice.'

If there's time, it's even better to voice the team's worry before having a separate meeting in a quiet room. It's less shocking and prepares the child's family to anticipate the worse news that will follow, the news that will change everything. As I sit in our meeting room and prepare what I'm going to say, I've been struck by the thought that in my mouth sit the words, waiting. They gather, gain shape and wait. Once those words are spoken, there will be such pain. The words are tiny daggers, laced with venom. They will fly to the hearts of the parents who sit with us and hurt them beyond all pain they have felt before.

I don't want to say anything, but I must go ahead and speak the dreadful words, to respect the child who is dying, and their family, so that they can share precious time with each other and fully understand that the end is soon.

It is in these moments that I feel closest to what unites us as humans. I draw on the pain of losing people I have loved. Each parent, no matter what has gone before, feels the intensity of this conversation. It is a meeting that will burn a hole in time, no matter how carefully and gently the chosen words are said. Afterwards, the time zone will shift from 'before we knew' to 'after we knew'. Every event in their lives will fall into one time zone or the other.

Although the news creates enormous pain, I believe people value honesty. The sharp blade of honesty is cushioned in the silk glove of authenticity and kindness. It is a paper-thin line between being explicit enough, yet stopping short of trampling on every dream and hope. There have been days when I've not got that balance right. There have been times when it feels cruel, no matter how hard you strive for kindness. From when I first began as a consultant in PICU, I recall a broken mother screaming at me over and over, 'Tell me how I can bury my child. How can I put him in a grave?' The image of this woman, whom we had torn apart with our words, sits heavily in my memory collage. Decades later, I wonder how she is and send her healing thoughts.

Everyone reacts differently to the news. So much depends on how the loss is projected onto everything that has already occurred in a person's life – which we can never know. We have cared for parents who have never seen the body of a loved one after death, who are terrified of what they might see. And we have cared for parents who are no strangers to dying, death and all its rituals. And every kind of reaction in between.

Margaret taught me a powerful lesson in exactly how merciless life can be for some people and the power of accepting suffering as a natural part of life.

Margaret was a young woman and a mother. She was a member of the Traveller community. She came into PICU the day after her baby, Paudie, was born by emergency caesarean section on the other side of the country. Her own mother was with her.

Paudie was critically ill, and we had no treatment that could help him. Sadly, he had been born with a severe abnormality of his chest, which affected both his lung and heart growth. He was supported fully with medication and intensive-care machines, but he was not going to survive. We held onto him as best we could overnight, until his mother could safely leave the maternity unit and see him.

Her mother pushed Margaret's wheelchair to the door of PICU and rang the bell. They had come to see Paudie together.

'Where's my baby?' Margaret asked.

We brought her to the side of his cot. She sat in silence staring at him. Paudie's nurse Maria told her that the PICU doctor would talk to her when she was ready.

'Is he going to live?' she asked.

I pulled up a chair and sat beside her. 'We're very worried he's not going to make it.' I paused, leaving silence hanging in the air between us. 'What do you think will happen?' I asked, after a minute or so.

'I think he's going to die, Doctor. Like the others did. Am I right?'

Margaret had borne five children and had just one small girl alive at home. Paudie was her fourth boy. Paudie's grandmother, Philomena, had given birth to twelve children, seven of whom had died in infancy. Cousins, aunts and sisters had the same story. A story of unbearable and unending loss.

We talked some more. Margaret showed me that evening she understood more about death and loss from her twenty-seven years of living than many people far older than her would ever know. Death was completely real to her. It was not something that came at the end of life: it was part of life, ever-present and already understood.

Her dignity in the moments of accepting Paudie's imminent death was immense. She simply bowed her head and closed her eyes. Her mother Philomena did the same. There was dignity, but there was also bitter resignation.

'I knew it,' Margaret stated, when I showed her the X-ray images of Paudie and explained his diagnosis. 'I knew he would be another one.'

A few hours later they asked for a priest. Our hospital chaplain came, and they thanked him many times for seeing them. Their gratitude was humbling. Paudie's father came in to see him and they baptised the baby together. Mother and daughter sat there all night, saying very little, and as dawn lit the window above Paudie's cot, he passed away. Their family waited outside the hospital. Margaret and Philomena did not want them present.

As is our custom we offered to help Margaret bring Paudie home, before they made their funeral arrangements. We have specific foldaway cots with an electric cooling mattress that we lend to bereaved families taking their dead baby home.

'I've no place for him,' she said.

'We'll mind him for you, keep him really safe here,' his nurse Niamh immediately reassured her.

Margaret nodded. 'We'll go now.'

Niamh tried to persuade them to stay a little longer, to wash Paudie and dress him. To take some rest and eat. She was troubled by their sorrowful acceptance and wanted to protect them in our haven. But with a stoicism that humbled each of us to the core, Margaret and Philomena left PICU, Paudie's fragile remains held in the arms of his nurse.

The bleak resignation with which they had lived those hours with us in PICU was profound.

50. The Bond That Is Created

'The battle of being mortal is the battle to maintain the integrity of one's life.'

Atul Gawande

As part of our training in medicine we were taught about the role of a physician. It meant having medical knowledge and using it to treat illness, guiding patients and advocating for them. How guidance is interpreted varies from doctor to doctor. In the more conservative past, doctors often believed that they knew what was best for their patients. In some situations, it even meant restricting access to personal information and issuing direction on family or social circumstances such as unplanned pregnancy. We are emerging from this paternalistic approach to see the patient as autonomous with the human right to respect as equal in every aspect of medical care.

As parents accompany their child through most of their contact with healthcare professionals, partnership in neonatal and paediatric medical care is well established. Although the emphasis is on the child, the relationships we build with their parents are a rich source of knowledge, inspiration and occasionally fun.

We admit a lot of newborns to the PICU, so we meet people who have just become parents. They are often wrestling with the emotions that come with being responsible for a baby. There can be confusion about illness and uncertainty about the future. It is a difficult place to begin a relationship. Many have a problem picked up on the scans their mother had during pregnancy and are electively delivered in a maternity unit as close to the children's hospital as possible. They often stay in the PICU for months, having surgery, which may be multiple, and recovering afterwards. A huge emphasis is placed on growth and development, in addition to recovery.

Important relationships are formed during that time. The most important relationship is the bonding between parents and their baby. It's not easy to bond with a baby that perhaps you can't cuddle or feed and who might be kept asleep for days. Placing emphasis on the connection that has already grown between parents and their baby before they were born can be helpful – re-framing the PICU stay in the newborn period as an interlude rather than an interrupted meeting for the first time.

Another important relationship is between the baby's parents and the multitude of team members in the PICU. Our nurses spend twelve hours of each shift at the side of the baby. They deliver specialised nursing care, and they support and care for baby and parents. They listen to worries and family stories, and they often go over medical information with parents, answering questions.

Adam and his dad Peter come to mind when I think of this key rapport between families and staff. From the day Adam arrived in the PICU, only a few hours old, Peter was a force of nature. Adam was incredibly sick and required a massive level of critical-care support. We were not sure he would make it to the first surgery he would need – but he wasn't stable or well enough to go through it yet. We were stuck in a long, hard climb to stability. Peter grilled us on every aspect. He had read a huge amount of material on Adam's illness before he was born and was ready to participate fully in every decision.

'Partnership in care' and 'shared decision-making' are terms we use in neonatal and children's medical care. Peter was the living embodiment of those terms, and he influenced my view on their importance. He was funny and often oddly relaxed in the PICU environment. He swore he had never crossed the door of a hospital before his wife became pregnant, though we asked him many times if he was sure he hadn't worked here in a past life.

Tiny Adam did not have a smooth path to recovery. There were a lot of dark days, when complications had occurred or treatment hadn't worked. Or yet another perilous surgery was needed. Each of these days had to be worked through together. We shared explanations with Peter and Amanda, Adam's mother. We had many discussions at Adam's bedspace and in multidisciplinary meetings, where staff and parents sit together and share concerns to forge a plan ahead, regrouping and trying to find another way out of the latest problem. Peter demanded openness at every point. 'I don't want bullshit,' he said, on the day Adam arrived, and that didn't change. He repeated the phrase whenever he thought we were trying to soften a piece of information.

It can be difficult for people to know and accept that there are days when their doctors don't know the next move. Children are individuals, with a very individual shape to their illnesses. When a new issue develops, there can be hours or days in which we use more tests or experience from other specialists to work out how significant the new issue is for that child. It creates even more fear in parents to hear, 'We don't know, but we will find out.'

It is a huge demand on a new relationship and another burden in an already demanding and emotionally charged situation. Complex illness in children asks so much from their parents. Although antenatal diagnosis can assist in preparing families for the road ahead, it provides only a rough map. It does not give insight into days of little hope, days of joy and months of uncertainty. Perhaps that is just as well: like many tough life experiences, we need to experience it for it to be meaningful.

Peter sometimes asked for time to go outside and look up stuff online. Occasionally he brought in a printed sheet of information, or questions to which he wanted answers. 'Just do your very, very best,' he would say with a smile, at the end of every discussion. Sometimes the smile was small, sometimes hardly there at all.

After many months, Adam went home. He was still on a schedule of drugs and feeds, underweight and delayed in meeting his developmental milestones. Such a tough start in life carries a heavy toll for a baby. On every visit back to the outpatient clinic, Peter brought Adam up to the

PICU to say hi and fill us in on the latest stories from their home. We heard about the dogs and the neighbours and, of course, what Adam was doing and how they were doing it with him. Whatever therapy had been prescribed or organised was always modified to fit in with their family life. That was Peter's way.

One afternoon without warning, after a long absence over the pandemic, Peter and Adam rang the bell of the PICU. A young slim boy, wearing a checked shirt and black jeans, walked in beside his dad. He held his dad's hand and looked around him with huge blue eyes. He looked like a thousand other boys his age.

It was Adam.

51. The Delicate Balance

'Learn how to be cursed, from him who taught you to love: the one hand brings the wound and the relief.'

Ovid

Over ten years in the PICU so much changed. My children grew up. They stopped wanting to come into work with me, content to hang out with their friends. Colleagues and friends, we all got older. There were lots of retirement lunches. We saw many parents and their children get older too. For many of them, getting older brought a whole new set of challenges. Families often had to fight for years to get basic services for their children, such as places in special schools and home nursing hours. Serious illness requiring readmission through the emergency department was a constant source of worry for parents of children with a life-limiting condition, as each hospital stay resulted in loss of function and independence. This anxiety could communicate itself as anger or frustration. It helped if we had a relationship already.

We did not always get along with parents as these are difficult relationships for everyone. Bella was Josh's mother, and we saw her a couple of times a year, when Josh had to be admitted to the PICU for management of a chest infection. He had a life-limiting genetic condition and many medical challenges associated with it. Bella was his carer and protector, as well as his mother. 'I love yis and I hate yis,' she would say, with a laugh. Despite their difficult life together, Bella laughed a lot.

Since we had first met, Bella's life had become even harder. Josh had grown larger, and his mobility had greatly suffered because of painful joints. He was a solid weight in a hoist and in a wheelchair. Bella resisted using a hoist as much as possible as she said it was quicker and easier to lift Josh. This was not easy, and we worried about their safety. Bella stooped and looked exhausted all the time. She fretted about his feeds and fought with our dietician regularly about changes to his feeding plan. Bella knew that when Josh became ill, he needed intensive care, but it was a demanding experience that never got any easier, no matter how well we all knew Josh and her.

Each day that Josh was with us in the PICU was another day on which Bella lost ground in the delicate balance she created when she had him at home. It took weeks to get him back into a schedule of sleep, activity and feeding well each time they left the hospital. Bella often mentioned the fight she had for community nursing help, supplies of incontinence wear and respite. 'Never mind a bloody wheelchair that fits him!' she would finish. Respite had stopped over the pandemic and Bella had not looked for it since. She didn't trust other people to care for Josh as she did. She was devoted to him, and his skin was always in perfect condition, his hair washed. Josh had thick, shiny black hair that would have made a teenage girl weep with jealousy. He adored his hair being washed and his head massaged, so Bella did this every day. She kept his hair quite long and fiercely resisted any suggestion of a trim. There was a special spark between Bella and one of the nursing shift leaders, Cathal, and he would tease her about Josh's hair and her devotion to it.

On one admission, Josh developed a pressure ulcer on one of his ankles. He had been sedated heavily for several days to tolerate a high level of support from the ventilator, as his lungs were flooded with infection. As he recovered, the ulcer grew in importance in Bella's mind. It was a significant complication, and we strive to avoid these from occurring. I sat with her and the lead nurse for the PICU and we talked about his skin care and how the ulcer had happened. We went around in circles for a bit, but I could see we were missing something. There was an air of frustration and rumbling fury in the room.

'I think you're very upset and angry with us that this has happened,' I said to her quietly.

She shook her head but said nothing. We sat in silence for a few minutes.

Then, for the first time, Bella cried. I was totally shocked. We had sat with her many times and talked about different unfortunate developments and setbacks. She had always been resolute in making choices for her son and in using facts to find a way forward. We had never seen her in tears before. But here she was, crying silently. About his skin. But it wasn't about his skin.

She found her words and spoke about the pain and guilt she felt for wanting to keep Josh with her all the time, for feeling she had let him down when he was critically ill. Her mind was besieged with self-doubt and recrimination about whether she had suctioned his airway enough; maybe she had run in his feed too fast; perhaps she could have done more to have him upright in his chair. Maybe she should have shouted louder for more help with him at home. Her tears of sadness and regret were for her actions, not ours. She said she didn't expect anything more of us, we were doing our best – but she could have done better. It was the lowest point in a line that had always been running downwards, despite Bella in her role as mother and carer, and her massive efforts.

I was called to an emergency but Cathal stayed in the conference room with Bella, reassuring her that no one could do better than she did. Bella then returned tearfully to Josh's room.

Our social worker made stellar efforts in the background over the next few weeks as Josh recovered, and their situation at home appeared a little more supported. Before discharge, we chatted to Bella about her wishes for Josh when he next became ill. She promised to think about a ceiling to medical interventions. None of the team wanted to see this beautiful boy sedated on a ventilator again any time soon, with all the problems that might quickly follow.

The thorny 'quality of life' question emerged. Carers see their loved ones in their worst health and their best. We see them only at their worst. What can be lost from the conversation is a snapshot of a child living well at home. In an ideal world, intensive-care staff would visit patients at home when they are well to learn and understand the wider perspective. The perspective of the child living well, recognising that their life may be short.

'I know what's best for Josh,' Bella said. 'I'll come back to you on this but give me time at home with him first.'

In the PICU we have to pause and consider what is in the best interests of a child – immediately and in the longer term. Every intervention we carry out comes at a human cost. Interventions, procedures, surgeries may bring hope and progress. But they also bring pain, confine a patient to a hospital bed and sometimes cause distressing problems. It can be difficult to initiate a conversation about the burden versus benefit of treatment.

We know that the experience of the person who spends all their time caring for the patient is central. Carers are far more than their role and what we see of their lives: they are fragile but strong people, with the right to be seen, heard and acknowledged. Receiving this recognition in healthcare grows trust and validates a life devoted to caring. This recognition is also needed from the state because it secures rights as a citizen. Honesty and willingness to listen to all views are the only ways to develop a relationship that is rich in trust. And time. Time is a friend in the relationship between a doctor and their patient. Josh's skin healed slowly, as his lungs did. We healed our friendship alongside.

On the day Josh went home – one more time, maybe – Bella brought him up to the PICU to say goodbye. She caught me by surprise, wrapping me in a big hug. It felt sisterly. Bella is a carer: a tiny word that means strength and goes far beyond five letters.

52. Darkness

'There is a black pit in the bottom of my soul that has no limit to its falling.'

Claire North

There is a side of the moon that no light ever reaches. Some sights we witness are filled with such filth and torn-apart flesh that nothing will ever seem right in the world again. Sometimes people ask, 'What's the worst thing you've ever seen?'

For me it will always be any incident in which a child has been abused.

There are people who inflict pain and damage beyond all comprehension on others, who cause suffering for babies and young children, then lie and deny it. There are painful fractures and abrasions on the tiny body of a five-week-old from someone lashing out in temper. There is the slow starvation and watchfulness seen in a neglected three-year-old. There are the swabs for sexually transmitted diseases, the bowel and genital injuries to be repaired surgically after the rape of a child. These children may be accompanied by parents, grandparents, older siblings. The emotional effects on everyone are destructive, as suspicion and blame corrode every interaction.

Mostly these images and memories I bury deep in a box inside my heart. I don't want to revisit them. Over time, the edges of the box have grown softer, the anguish ebbing to a dull ache. As ever, it's wisest to summon the memory of what was good or right. I try to leave a horrifying scene with one good thing. It could be a lesson to return to later, a kind word from a colleague, pride in doing my best, a magnificent dawn . . . anything. Something good that I can savour as I think of the patient, saying their name in my mind and thanking them.

In the swirl of darkness, I reach into the box and recall Brenda, one of the PICU nurses, and I standing in a room with baby John. He had been brought to the hospital too late after his injuries had been inflicted. We were powerless to stop his spirit leaving. His clotting system was so broken at that stage that he was bleeding freely from his nose, eyes, everywhere. His dark curls were matted with blood. John fought to live, scrabbling at the air. His parents were not present and could not be.

Brenda focused on giving John pain relief, but it was horribly distressing. As his little body relaxed towards death, we agreed that we could not accept him passing without being held and loved. Brenda sat in the reclining chair that parents usually use, and I lifted John onto her lap. Her scrubs quickly became stained red, but she did not appear to notice. Instead, Brenda cradled John close to her and whispered, 'You are loved now, you are special, John, go with love, John, go with love, go with love.' I had never heard those words said like that before, or since. The capacity of that young woman, not yet a mother, to immerse John instinctively in her loving embrace restored a sliver of goodness to that dreadful night.

We were joined by the nursing shift leader, Libby and we clung to each other in silence, not sure if we could ever walk out of that room and be OK again. It was some time before I had the strength to leave it and phone the coroner, partly because I was so distraught by what had been done to John – he had been beaten so badly by someone who was meant to be caring for him – and partly because as soon as I made that phone call, I knew John would lose his humanity.

He would no longer be the tiny boy who deserved unconditional love but who had not received it. He would become a legal case, a process, with documents and reports. For some of the reports, even his name would be obscured, and he would become an initial or a number. It is events that are inflicted on children like John and the way their personhood subsequently disappears that explains my complete absence of religious faith, although I deeply envy those who have that sanctuary.

Several hours later, when John had gone to the mortuary, I saw Brenda back in the same room. She had had a shower and changed her scrubs, and her damp hair hung down in a braid, making the back of her tunic dark with moisture. She was busy preparing equipment at the bedspace, setting up for a new admission, who would arrive in the next few minutes. As I walked past, she gave me a brave smile. It was the shared smile of 'we'll be OK' that we give each other when there are no words to capture how demolished we feel. Brenda looked utterly hollowed out. In solidarity, we were human husks, dry and barren inside.

Somehow, she would find the humanity and care to give the next child who would occupy that room. Their parents would not know what had happened there in the hours before their child was admitted. Brenda's strength and skill are to be prized, and for that reason alone it is a memory to be preserved.

I could never forget John. Or all the others. In paediatric intensive care, we observe the consequences of what adults do, or do not do. The children we admit who have been injured by an adult touch our hearts in a way that isn't possible with any other child. Love and protection are two powerful reflexes that spring into force among staff in this situation. We treat the consequences and report the medical findings as we work our way through the debris left behind. We document what we find, collate our clinical information, refer to state agencies and write reports for any legal proceedings that follow. Each of these tasks is done with protection at its core.

The dark side of paediatrics is rare. We will never know the full picture. That can be difficult to accept. There will never be an opportunity to understand why a human would hurt another in this way. Most of us will not attend any court proceedings or even hear of them happening. Several years later, there may be a brief court report in a newspaper, and we will wonder it that is justice for 'our' child. A child's need for safety, support and treatment extends far outside what we can do over a short number of days or weeks in the intensive-care unit, or on the paediatric wards.

There are external psychological supports available for us, although mostly it is the immediate early support and listening from colleagues that is most helpful. These are not stories that can be brought home. We care for the children with love and skill for as long as they are with us. One good thing that many of us take away is a hunger and gratitude for love and safety in our own lives.

This darkness is by far the most haunting element of our work, and peace or sleep is not easily found afterwards. The elements that I have found lead to some ease in my heart are the love we show the child, a focus on who helped at the time and, lastly, how we carried on to love more children. This is why Brenda and Libby and all our PICU team shine bright in my memory. They are the lighthouse, shining across the dark seas.

53. To Keep Hope

'All human wisdom is summed up in two words: wait,
and hope.'

Alexandre Dumas

One Friday morning my husband was away for work. I raced
the children into their clothes and down the stairs for
breakfast. We had a mission. Friday was Irish spelling test
day, and we had to get the spellings letter-perfect before I
left for the hospital. Between mouthfuls of toast, the words
were practised. Barry was brilliant with the children and
their schoolwork, patiently going over their lessons until
they knew the words. It was a bit more chaotic when I was
leading the charge. The children knew this and took full
advantage.

When I arrived into morning handover in the PICU, I
described the kitchen scene for the team, who laughed and
immediately recounted their own tales of spelling tests and
learning times-tables in school and in a hurry before a test.

We moved on to discuss one of our most recent admissions, Maeve. She was our little princess from the Gaeltacht.

She spoke only Irish. In her four years of life, she had never left the far northern edge of Ireland, until she needed urgent medical treatment. She had been in hospital for a few days having tests done, before going to the operating room for major surgery. Her problem was rare, and a big team of surgeons had collaborated on the day of the operation. That surgery had been longer and even more complicated than anticipated, and Maeve had come to us in the PICU afterwards. She had lost a lot of blood, and it was proving challenging to source the correct blood products for her as she had a more unusual blood type. Nothing seemed straightforward for this new little patient.

We settled Maeve into her room, on a significant amount of medication and mechanical support for her organs. This first night would be extremely important in establishing her on the road to recovery. That was when we met Noirin, Maeve's mother. She was one of the strongest people I've met, in a world where inner strength is forged in the fires of fear and fight for life. Noirin's husband had lost his life the year before in a tragic fishing accident, when the boat he was on sank in the wild sea off the coast. His brother, too, had drowned. When Noirin told us this story, we remembered it from the news updates, as it had taken some time to find their bodies. Now her precious only child, Maeve, was critically ill.

The tragedy that had been far away on the radio for all of us was now heavy in the air of the room where Maeve lay. We desperately wanted to give Noirin hope. In fact, the opposite occurred. She gave us an example of the power of hope and patience.

Noirin was the living embodiment of optimism that everything would be better if we could all get through this. She dragged hope out of us and was not taking no for an answer. She entertained everyone in the PICU for weeks, reading poetry aloud, singing *sean-nós* and telling stories. She was a diminutive woman, old beyond her years, quick-witted and wise. Loss has that effect on some people – it allows them to go deeper into living, deeper into thinking and feeling than others not marked by such sadness. If someone had said that Noirin was a spirit, or a fairy, I think we would have believed it.

She sat every day beside Maeve, watching her child sleep and watching the staff caring for Maeve. As I expressed my sympathies to her one day on the loss of her husband, she calmly told me she wished she had had the opportunity to sit with him and listen to his sleeping breath as he died. 'Being with Maeve in the PICU holds no fear for me,' she continued, as she knew that this was a hopeful place, a refuge of hope. *Dóchas.* She explained that it was the uncertainty of 'after the PICU' that distressed her. Would 'after the PICU' see Maeve and Noirin at home together or Noirin alone? That was her fear.

Her hope was tested. Maeve made initial progress and began to wake up and recognise her mother. But those early days were followed by a leak in the wall of her bowel, which made Maeve critically ill for a second time. Before she had really recovered from the first surgery, she was heading back to the operating room for more intervention.

For a second time after major surgery, Maeve's kidneys stopped working. We set up for dialysis to support her kidneys and to wait until all the medications and organ rest worked. And hoped.

Then Maeve started having seizures. That phone call in the middle of the night saying she had had a brief seizure brought our spirits low. 'Dispirited' is the perfect word for how we felt at the dawning realisation that everything was not going to be OK. Noirin sank low into her chair and sobbed without stopping that day.

Once lost, hope and the will to live seldom return.

We scanned Maeve's brain to make sure she had not had a bleed or collection of infection develop there. There was nothing to see, other than her swollen brain. We treated her with medication to stop the seizures and rest her brain completely. Her little body was receiving dozens of medicines, each one in powerful doses. Every medicine has its own potential side-effects, and interactions with each other must be anticipated and managed.

The waiting began again. No one ever talks about how difficult and painful waiting is. Noirin guided the whole team through those boiling dark seas by resuming her campaign of hope. It is simplistic to say that our job in healthcare is to use knowledge and experience to treat a child, and the job of the parents is to love and keep hope. But many times, this is the situation. In paediatric medicine, that relationship often shifts, and we share love, experience and hope freely with everyone around the bed of a sick child.

We were conscious that Noirin was carrying the heavy burden of knowing that bad things do happen, bad things happen to good people, and perhaps without warning. The muscles used to lift spirits each day were achy and strained by evening.

After three long days, Maeve's condition began to improve. Oh, the delight we shared in counting drops of urine as her kidneys began to function again. We smiled with pleasure, sharing the news of falling white cells and decreasing heart medicines with Noirin. She asked questions about Maeve's X-rays and her breathing support. She had asked very little before this, but she had been listening to every word. The hours speeded up as we entered the most wonderful time in a child's admission to critical care – recovery.

Maeve gradually woke up and we saw no more of the convulsions that had scared everyone so much. She came off all the machines, one by one. It took much patience to encourage her gut to work again, and her little mouth was sore and thirsty. She did not complain much, even when we lifted her out of bed and onto her mother's lap, drips and monitors trailing like vines around her skinny frame.

During these mellow weeks of recovery Noirin apologised profusely that she had only taught Maeve to speak Irish. A wild blend of languages flowed through the room, Maeve cared for by nurses and doctors from around the world. It is extraordinary how love and care can smooth the wrinkles of language differences. *'Táim ceart go leor'* – I'm OK – and *'go hiontach'* – that's great – joined the vocabulary of the PICU staff no matter where they were from.

Maeve survived two life-threatening events. Noirin survived, clinging to love and almost losing hope. Hope is the air we breathe, each breath expecting the best.

The end of hope is devastating.

54. Sharing the Day

'If everything around seems dark, look again: you may be the light.'

Rumi

Caught in the middle of an interminable bad dream, any parent would be forgiven for not seeing left or right of them. Their focus is their child and their child's recovery, followed by whatever is happening at home. But parents give each other tremendous encouragement. Ben's family were the absolute best when it came to helping other scared parents find their way around PICU life.

Ben was a patient with us for many months, recovering from serious burns to his face, neck and chest. His dad Rory and mum Ava spent the first two weeks in a haze of shock, surgeries and setbacks. As they emerged from the shock, they entered the dull, heavy waters of slow recovery. It was in these later weeks that we got to know them better. They were helpers and had a keen eye for other people in the PICU who needed support.

We had a medical student assigned to the PICU. He

disappeared into Ben's room each day and didn't emerge for hours, beguiled by stories about parenting and children. Ava encouraged the student to practise asking her questions, which was comical and endearing to listen to, as I heard her patiently correcting him by saying, 'Ah, no, love, you can't ask it like that!' When I thanked her for giving our medical student so much of her time, she replied, 'Sure I like doing it, and it makes the time pass.'

One evening on call, we admitted a young baby from the emergency department with an infection of her lungs. We brought her and her terrified mother up to the PICU, asking the mother to wait in the parents' sitting room while we started her baby on help to breathe and made a more detailed assessment.

Margo, the baby's PICU nurse, reminded me to go out about an hour later to chat to the new admission's mother, Beth. I found her sitting with Ben's family. Rory was in full flight, explaining to the young mother why she was waiting outside the PICU. Ava had her arm around the woman's shoulders, reassuring her that everything would be OK. We stood for a moment in the doorway and watched the scene. It was touching to see one stranger's kindness to another. 'Hi, Beth, we'll sit down next door and go through some pieces of information with you, then bring you in to your baby. She's stable now,' Margo said.

'Do you see?' said Ava. 'It's all under control.' I grimaced to myself at this: control and stability in intensive care can change in a second. But I smiled and thanked Ava and Rory for looking after Beth.

The support didn't stop there. Looking back, I realise that

support goes both ways: Ava and Rory were helped by the help they gave. They opened their hearts and gave generously of their time. For the next two weeks they chatted to Beth, whom they had taken under their wing. I frequently saw them checking in on her and her child before they left in the evening.

When I left for home in the evenings, I observed them sitting outside the hospital chatting to other parents. As I cycled past the group, they gave me cheery waves goodnight. A community grows in the uncomfortable grounds of a hospital, bright poppies in the cracks between the concrete slabs. During Ben's stay, his parents put out their hands to other parents sharing a difficult chapter in their lives.

The bond between parents of sick children is unique. They share an experience that is difficult to explain to people outside a children's hospital. Parents have often spoken about the pressure from home to give an optimistic update each day, some tiny gem of good news. But there are days when there isn't any good news. And days when there is nothing to say or no energy to say it.

Ava spoke about the conversations they all had in the evenings, outside the PICU. 'We know all of you, your habits and the way things work!' She laughed cheekily, and I didn't ask any more.

The parents also share the knowledge that there are good days and bad days. There are days that are just disappointing and dull, and days of exhausted relief. Some families keep in touch after discharge, through Facebook groups or other platforms, but most do not. Warm and supportive to each other at the time of the admission, it is equally therapeutic to close the chapter.

55. One Mother to Another

'Youth fades, love droops; the leaves of friendship fall; a mother's secret hope outlives them all.'
Oliver Wendell Holmes

I can't lie and say that my experience of working with children didn't change how I parented. Even when my children had grown into teenagers, I cut their grapes in two and warned them not to put small objects into their mouths. They thought these admonishments were funny and would tease me as they got older. On the plus side, I couldn't bring myself to chastise them to study harder or go out with their friends less. The big picture of how life could change in a second was never far from my mind. It was not possible to view childhood in any other way. We relished the fun. But we knew we were lucky.

We also knew that our family had been tested already and could not be certain we would survive another blow. It made me cautious.

We drew strength from children like Andrej, and his parents, Eric and Violetta. She was one of those mothers who cling to their children with the ferocity of a tiger. She didn't have much spoken English but instead had the most expressive eyes and hands I've ever come across. Her toddler, Andrej, came to the PICU from another hospital. He'd had a coughing event a few days earlier and Violetta had noticed he was eating less and becoming lethargic. Most worryingly, he was now drooling and had stopped speaking. An X-ray of his neck and chest in the emergency department where Violetta had brought him showed a tiny disc-shaped object in the centre of his chest. It appeared that Andrej had swallowed an old coin, which had lodged there and was likely causing damage. When he arrived in the PICU he was combative and scared, so we left him sitting on Violetta's lap and gently moved around him getting him ready for surgery to remove the coin.

The ear, nose and throat surgeon came over and we had a discussion with Violetta and her husband Eric about the plan. The surgeon was very concerned about what he might find when he inserted a long slim camera into Andrej's breathing and swallowing tubes, the trachea and the oesophagus, to locate the coin. One of the cardiac surgeons joined us by phone to add some thoughts.

Violetta patiently held Andrej upright to her own body as he dozed, dirty secretions oozing from his mouth and nose. She waited for Eric to translate and explain the plan, her large brown eyes fixed on our faces as we spoke. When everyone seemed clear on our next steps, we gave them a few minutes to call their families while the anaesthesiologist, Terence, came over from the operating room to assess and transport Andrej for surgery. Terence immediately understood the mix of emotions in the room: fear, dismay and relief. To some smiles from the nurses and the porter, Terence helped Violetta climb up onto the patient trolley, still clutching Andrej. 'Sure, we'll all go together,' he said, with wisdom and kindness.

Andrej was gone for hours. Occupied with a full PICU, I realised how long they had been away only as we prepared to begin our handover for the night shift. I walked over to the operating room and saw rushing staff, heard calls for more equipment and more blood products. My heart sank. I insinuated myself as far as I could into the room, and Terence spotted me and came over.

'The coin had completely corroded and worn through Andrej's oesophagus. All the tissues around were filthy and damaged, including the delicate supporting tissues and blood vessels around his heart, trachea and lungs. Believe it or not,' he said, waving a hand across the busy room, 'we're a lot more stable now, and should be over to you in another hour or so.' I thanked him and returned to start the difficult explanation for Eric and Violetta, who paced the floor in the parents' lounge. Andrej would need the very best of good fortune to survive such severe damage and infection.

The first few days were rough. Andrej had to remain completely still under a blanket of sedation and medicines to stop his muscles moving. He looked dreadful. Dark brown smelly secretions continued to pour from his nose and mouth, and he became bloated with fluid. His appearance was the very definition of sickness. Despite how distressing this was for his parents and the nurses caring for Andrej, we were delighted that his heart and kidneys held firm. He continued to develop a horrible pneumonia in both lungs.

The lining around them had been damaged so they blew air bubbles through a multitude of drains that stood, like soldiers, around his bed.

If Andrej survived these initial rocky days, he would not be able to swallow and feed normally for months, so a feeding tube had been brought out by the surgeons through the wall of his tummy. Andrej clung to life in the same way he had clung to his mother. On the second evening, after nursing handover, his night nurse, Hayley, asked me to meet Violetta at the door as she returned and distract her for a few minutes.

'What are you going to do?' I asked Hayley.

'I want to give Andrej a really good clean,' she answered straight away. 'Especially his mouth, that's really important for his mum,' she went on.

'Why is his mouth so important?' I wondered aloud.

'Suzanne, mothers always notice their child's mouth first. It's the first thing they look at, and it's upsetting for a mum to see her child's mouth dry or cracked or not clean,' Hayley explained to me. In that moment, I was moved with respect for our nurses who understand these basic human needs and attend to them by giving care the importance it deserves.

Violetta sat each day and waited patiently. She played music for Andrej and often sang and hummed along with it. One day as I stood at Andrej's bed, she looked at me with consternation. 'Will he talk?' she asked, fear filling her face as some of the possible consequences had begun to arrive in her mind.

'We hope so,' I said, with a smile.

'Thank you,' she replied.

'I am very sure that Andrej can hear your music and your songs,' I said. 'That is very good for him,' I continued, and gave her a small hug as I left. The PICU nurses worried about how little Violetta seemed to sleep and eat, and in the background, they minded her as they cared for all the patients. When Violetta arrived early in the morning, a kind healthcare assistant draped a blanket around her shoulders as she sat, and later snoozed. Small meals seemed to make their way to her and I'm not quite sure how that happened, but I knew it was done with love and the solidarity of mothers. Too many times to count, I have noticed the nurses squirrelling away food for a mother. Eric worked long shifts in a factory on the other side of the country, so we didn't see him so much, but the day never ended without Violetta holding her mobile phone up to one of the PICU doctors, with the words 'Please, talk to Eric', before she herself said goodnight and thank you to everyone.

Andrej was gradually allowed to wake up and move. The swelling receded and he began to look better. His pain management was a major challenge for us over the first weeks of recovery, as he had such a complicated injury from the coin.

He returned to the operating room several times for repair of tissues or replacement of drains in the space around his lungs. His bowels stopped working for a while, which introduced new difficulty when nutrition was needed more than ever. Each episode set the clock back to zero, with worry and a new cycle of pain. The story sounds incredibly bleak now, but there was never a loss of optimism among the team that Andrej would get through this awful experience. Each day we catalogued the list of obstacles that faced him, the tasks still to be completed and the possible complications that might hide around the next corner, like masked highwaymen.

It's difficult to explain why some patients are surrounded by this continuing positivity and others are not. Experience suggests that because Andrej was a healthy child when this event occurred, because we knew the cause, the potential problems, and he had the love and care of so many people, he would most likely survive. And he did. An experience like this can be very good for the staff, healing some of the personal and professional distress that critical care can bring.

Andrej was discharged to the ward after eighteen weeks in the PICU, a noisy, grumpy toddler who would need months of follow-up. We transferred him back to the children's ward in the hospital closest to where he lived with his parents, so that Eric could finally spend more time with him.

Three years later Eric and Violetta sent a card to the PICU staff, and a photo of Andrej in his school uniform. Blue-collared T-shirt, grey sweater and a big smile, Andrej was starting primary school. He held a colourful book, and Eric's hand on his shoulder was visible to the side – probably to keep Andrej still for the moment it took to snap the picture. It made me laugh to imagine the scene. His blond curls lay thick around his ears, but if you peered very closely at the picture, it was possible to see a few small scars on the side of his neck. 'Thank you,' said the card that accompanied the photo. 'Andrej has a sister now. Her name is Victoria.' The second picture in the envelope was of Violetta proudly cradling a small baby in her arms.

I felt a rush of love and protection for her, one mother to another, as I looked at the image. 'Thank you,' I said silently back to her.

56. Remembrance

*'Knowing your own darkness is the best method for dealing
with the darkness of other people.'*

Carl Jung

Each November we gather to read aloud the names of
children and babies who have died in the hospital and write
their names in the book of remembrance. It is a day that
honours the lives of the children and emotionally validates
the love and experience of care in which we have all played
a part. The event is held on a Saturday in the city centre,
at the darkest time of the year. It is just as the Christmas
lights appear. It is bittersweet.

I recall arriving one year, the venue already thronged
with people. June, from the pastoral-care team, was
buzzing around handing out name badges and goody-bags
for the children. There were plenty of smiles and warm
embraces. Our PICU administrator, Avril, was there
helping families settle in. Like all the staff, she had felt
drawn to this day and left her boys at home to join in. I
waved at familiar faces left and right of me as I hung up

my heavy winter coat, a knot of anticipation and tension in my chest.

Suddenly I was hugged from behind by a tall woman in glasses. 'I'm Kate!' she says. 'I just wanted to say thank you for everything.' She was wearing a red festive sweater, and it was difficult to place her in my mind initially. She pulled a man beside her closer and said, 'And you remember Andy too?' And then I did. I remembered them both and their delicate daughter Eabha who had lost her fight to overcome extreme prematurity and infection. Now that I had located them in my memory, I could remember them devastated in Eabha's room, cradling their daughter as she left them. Their pleas, their tears, their acceptance.

'Thank you for this day,' said Andy, with the same serious manner I recalled from months earlier. That seemed to be enough for them to say, and they dipped their heads with sad smiles and headed into the crowd. It felt good to see them together, holding hands.

As I crossed the room, I met Majella and Nick with their now ten-year-old son Ollie and six-month-old Ella. We hugged as they showed me their beautiful daughter, who was sleeping in her buggy. It was joyful. They all looked so healthy and content and spoke warmly of the opportunity to come to the ceremony. They had driven down from the north, up early in frosty weather, and had put in a few hours of Christmas shopping first.

'We knew we wouldn't be able to hit the shops after this,' said Nick, waving his hand across the big conference space in Dublin Castle, which was now filled with families and hospital staff enjoying each other's company. He was right. The air was swirling with emotion.

As the crowd took their seats, I sat towards the front feeling nervous. In my hand I held a list of the names of children who had died in the PICU that year. Fifty-two names. More than any other task in front of me, I wanted to do a good job. I wanted to walk up steadily to the lectern and read each name slowly, pronounce it correctly and give it the dignity and weight it deserved. To hold the family of each child in their own moment, as they stood into the aisle and walked up to hang a star on the huge tree at the top of the room. It felt like seconds, passing over hours, as we shared memories. The value of a name being said aloud was dear to my heart.

When I read out the name of Majella and Nick's toddler son, who had lost his life in a tragic accident, I saw Majella break into tears as she stood up. She clutched baby Ella in her arms as Nick took big brother Ollie's hand and they made their way up. Ollie stood on his tippy toes and hung a silver star with his brother's name 'Harry' on it, high on a branch that stood pointing upwards. Then they folded each other into a hug.

In my mind, I could see them in that same hug almost a year earlier, at the bed of her son Harry, as his spirit left the body of this curious and beloved boy. Majella had been pregnant at the time and the poignancy of new life growing as young life was suddenly stolen away seemed to add to the sadness. Now the new life seemed to ease the pain a fraction.

We were there to honour the lives of children and the privilege of having been involved in their care. In the background, I also brought the loss of my daughter to the ceremony of remembrance. Each year I imagined writing 'Beatrice' in the book, saying her name proudly and hanging her star on the tree. The families I have met over three decades have shown me that there is no weakness in vulnerability. Quite the opposite is true. Wearing the fragility of our humanity close to the surface in every interaction opens the door to a richer relationship with those around you, and with yourself. I believe many of us as staff brought our personal experiences of loss to those special days.

Through my daughter, I learnt so much. I was so fortunate to be able to make a choice and act with renewed purpose in the years after her brief life and death. At the core of existentialism are freedom and agency. She gifted me both. But even before her, there were many other individuals. My sister Louise, baby Alannah and her devastated parents ensured that I would become a doctor for sick children. Ever after I would strive to acquire skills and knowledge to help parents in pain. Deep down, I wanted never to feel incapable of supporting such a distressed young couple again.

Mrs Johnson and my grandfather showed me the reasons why these skills and knowledge would make a difference to people, to myself and my own family. But they also asked for reflection. And humanity. I saw that putting the needs of another ahead of your own could bestow knowledge and contentment on your heart.

However, my profession and its demands took a tremendous toll on my family and my relationships. As an intern, I missed the christening of my godchild. I was almost unknown in my children's schools, and parent-teacher meetings were few. I failed them many times by walking out of the door to return to work when on call. My son Arthur crying at the front door once wailed at me, 'Can no other doctor go?'

Perhaps another doctor could have gone. I realise how being a doctor fulfilled some of my own need to be valued. I see it, and it is my only source of regret.

Skye and her mother Josie helped me to understand the effects of being moved from foster care to foster care, how being homeless seeps into every cell and colours every interaction, no matter how supportive. A baby admitted to intensive care with an infected nappy rash because her homeless mother walks the streets with her all day sums up every injustice that some children and their parents experience in our society. That situation can never be right. We must not stay silent when we see such cruelty.

Recognising the gifts that people offer each other amid terror has been a wonderful lesson. The gift of a listening ear or of silence. The gift of learning and years of dedicated training that can make a child recover from an injury or illness and go home. The unbridled generosity of giving breast milk to a stranger's baby, or blood to a child having surgery, or heart valves or kidneys and a liver to a child who will survive, when yours will not.

There is a circle of giving around us that often we do not notice. When we notice it, we see it everywhere, and it becomes easy to step into it and play a tiny part in the circle. Awareness of it has the capacity to restore faith in the goodness of humanity. Lots of parents become involved in fundraising, advocacy or volunteer support following their own experiences with a sick child. This is no coincidence: within the act of giving, there is compassion.

Sam, Anna, Patrick and their families faced hurdles during their lives that I would not have believed possible had I never worked with children. They faced these obstacles every day. Physical and intellectual disability arises from a thousand different causes. It is not an option that people have selected: it is a part of them. There are many other parts of equal importance.

Disability is incredibly common, which makes it even more difficult to accept that our society sees it as an afterthought. 'This requires additional resources' or 'We must now make this thing we've already decided accessible to people who will struggle to use it' are attitudes that will not get us to where we need to be.

There is a fundamental need for humans to be together when life ebbs away. Separation at this significant time is felt deeply. Baby Grace died without her mother. There have been many more. I received the message that my daughter was dying while my husband and children were in another country. We were lucky to be together and hold her as she passed.

What we say to each other matters. Rebecca, Jonathan and hundreds more have taught me this. Comments made by staff caring for my daughter and me wounded me deeply. They were not intended to harm, but because of my heightened state of anxiety and fear, the words felt harsh and judgemental. They reverberated around my head for months after, giving my dark thoughts a focus to cleave to.

Words are incredibly powerful. They should be valued in their weight, like the most precious metals. Built into their meanings, their sound and the tone in which they are said, there is a force that can literally change how people think, feel and act. Each word exists with silence around it. We can choose silence in the sentence rather than speak a hasty word.

My experience has shown me that emotions influence the decisions we make, just as the outcome of those decisions influences the emotions that follow. The expression of emotion is not dangerous. Dissent and anger are human responses to attack. As healthcare staff we frequently do not anticipate the anger that families and patients feel, because we do not see or understand the perceived attack. Although my body will still react physiologically to an angry person, I now remind myself of the deep pain they are experiencing. Containment until some emotion ebbs away is important for everyone's safety, followed by communication to find out and address the true cause.

People from all backgrounds cherish an opportunity to speak and to be listened to with respect. Curiosity for the lives of people, for what is important to them, is a natural way to draw out hopes and fears. The common experience of caring for children is a foundation upon which an understanding can be built. Even more so, the common experience of being a child, needing love and attention, is inside all of us. As a doctor, I found it possible to connect to the child inside people, and inside me.

I made many mistakes, some because I didn't know enough. Others were because I believed I knew a lot. There were mistakes of judgement, of situations and of individuals. Writing these stories that go back over thirty years has shown me that there was greater good than harm. There are thousands more stories. Far from being angelic or perfect, we hope each day to do a good job that helps someone. From this there is much inner nourishment.

Sophie, Paudie and Grace were babies we could not help. Accepting as a doctor that some illnesses cannot be mended is difficult. Our entire education is focused on collecting knowledge and using information to repair and replace. Our patients and their parents are frequently wiser on the reality that some situations are irreparable, as they feel it and know it in an ancient way that is within all of us. It is possible to nurture that sense and give it space. My granddad told me this.

There have been occasions where we have done more interventions than we should have. In those decisions there was a child who lived uncomfortably for a day longer or a week longer because of our ego and desire to help. When I learnt to accept and embrace the end of life, my ability to work as a doctor improved. When I finally relented and allowed this wisdom into my own family loss, healing began.

Hope is at the door of every room in the PICU, a gossamer-thin curtain swaying in the breeze. In almost every conversation we have with families, we return to hope. We hope for a successful surgery, for a day of stability, for a positive test result. We hope for recovery.

Early in my time as a consultant I took all hope from a family during a difficult discussion. I did it deliberately because I thought it would help their understanding of the grave situation. It was a mistake: it damaged the trust between us, and I was never so harsh again with anyone. I learnt that it is possible to explain a devastating situation that will not recover and still leave space for hope. Because hope can come in and change everything. Although a baby dies, there can be hope in a peaceful death together, in the continuing bonds after death, in a couple who love each other, in a family who speaks the name of their baby daily. And so many other little and not so little ways that we may not know.

Narrative is a silver thread running throughout this tapestry. A glint in the light, it is glimpsed at important times in our lives. We weave this magnificent cloth together, telling tales of great courage and of a sense of rightness. It gifts reassurance that we know where we are. Love, hope, family and security are our cardinal touch points, and our shared narrative ensures that we always stay close to these. We witness the moment when a family open a new chapter in their story. It is awe-inspiring. They select the important words for them, and their story cascades around those first words. It holds them steady for many years.

Presence is the soil in which these seeds flourish. There have been days when the most important action I took was to sit beside a distressed parent and listen to them. Just sitting in silence for hours beside another person. Afterwards I questioned if I could have done more. I believe now that it was enough. The life of medicine is not knowledge: it is experience.

These are my reflections as I sit with parents at the remembrance ceremony. We mirror each other, and it feels safe.

They are my tribe.

This tender gathering of hurting humans feels like home.

57. She Loves the Swing

'For what pleasure can compare the pleasure of bringing joy and hope to other hearts? The more we make others happy, the greater will be our own happiness and the deeper our sense of having served humanity.'

Shoghi Effendi

After work, on a warm summer's evening, I took our youngest boy, Charles, to the park. It was just the two of us. My older children were now all teenagers and preferred the company of their friends. Charles loved the playground and was determined to master the monkey bars, so he grabbed any opportunity to practise.

We cycled up the quiet streets to the park. It felt like the rest of the city had left to take holidays. We had the playground to ourselves, which delighted Charles. A discarded sweater hung on the railings near the gate. The bins brimmed with the ends of picnics.

I sat on a bench near the climbing frames and watched him. The sun hung low, flitting through the branches of the trees around us. It was almost dusk. My mind played over the day at work. It had been a gentle one.

'Look, Mum!' called Charles, as he hung upside-down on the climbing frame.

'I see you!' I called back.

Out of the corner of my eye I saw a woman walk through the red metal gate of the playground. She had a small girl on a scooter with her. The young woman lifted the child into a swing and pushed her high in the air. She shouted with excited giggles. It was the most beautiful sound.

There was something familiar about the woman, but I couldn't quite place her in my mind. I went back to cheering Charles on in his fearless climbing feats. Behind me, I could hear chatter from the little girl.

Across the dusky park, a bell rang.

'Mum, the park keeper is coming!' shouted Charles. He found the idea of a park keeper throwing us out of the park both terrifying and wonderful.

'We can stay on a bit longer,' I said mischievously. 'Let's wait until he comes up to the playground.'

I knew Charles wouldn't last, as the bell rang closer to us. Through the trees, I could see the park keeper approaching.

'Right, matey, let's head for home,' I said to my darling boy.

We happily turned towards the gate.

The woman stood waiting there, holding the little girl's hand. 'Jessica loves the swing,' she said to me, with a broad smile. 'It's impossible to get her off it.'

'Oh, I know that one,' I replied.

'I have you to thank for it!' said the woman. 'You looked after her when she was sick as a baby.'

'Oh, my goodness, I wouldn't have known her,' I exclaimed, 'but I did kind of recognise you.'

'You help so many people, it would be impossible to remember everyone,' she said. 'But we remember you. Thank you.'

As the park keeper called across to us that it was time to leave, Charles tugged at my arm. 'C'mon, Mum!'

I said goodbye to the woman and her daughter, and we went home. We stopped for an ice cream on the way, leading Charles to declare it 'a great day'.

My heart was full and light.

Critically sick children and their families teach us how to live in the moment, how to die, how to accept and how to extract meaning from every moment we love and live together. There is a quiet strength to be found in each other's stories. We are not alone. We don't overcome grief; together, we weave it into something meaningful.

We distil that pain into hope, and it becomes a poem that never leaves your lips.

Acknowledgements

This book is about children and how loving a child can change our way of living.

I'd like to acknowledge the children and their families whom I have had the joy of meeting and caring for. Their courage left an indelible mark on me, which I have tried to honour but know that it would be impossible to replicate.

Thanks to my agent, Conor Nagle, for his enthusiasm from day one. Thanks to Ciara Considine and Stephen Riordan in Hachette Books Ireland for their unending patience and belief that this would happen. I am grateful to Hazel Orme for the time she took with this book – her suggestions helped a lot.

Thank you to all the healthcare professionals whom I have worked with over the years, especially the nursing staff in paediatric intensive care – their kindness has taught me and held me. This book is written with you in my heart.

And to my colleagues, who have given me huge personal and professional support.

Thanks to our family GP Dr Eamon Kelly who sowed the early seeds of possibility. Those seeds were nourished by dozens of teachers and mentors that I was fortunate to meet.

A note of recognition for Mary McCarthy, freelance journalist, and Tom Coogan, editor in the *Irish Independent*, who encouraged me to share the experience of working in healthcare, as a doctor, a widow, a patient and a mother. They both helped me to move writing muscles that I hadn't flexed in a long while.

Thanks to my children, Arthur, Estella, Dorothea, Beatrice and Charles. They have been my guide. And my late husband, Barry, who was a tower of strength throughout and is missed every day.

Deep gratitude to my parents, Ann and Brian. They have always been kind and wise.

To my circle of family and friends, you are just brilliant, thank you.